A COURSEBOOK

ON

SCIENTIFIC AND PROFESSIONAL WRITING

IN

SPEECH-LANGUAGE PATHOLOGY

A COURSEBOOK
ON
SCIENTIFIC AND
PROFESSIONAL WRITING
IN
SPEECH-LANGUAGE PATHOLOGY

M. N. Hegde, Ph.D.

California State University-Fresno

SINGULAR PUBLISHING GROUP, INC.

SAN DIEGO, CALIFORNIA

Singular Textbook Series

Series Editor: M. N. Hegde, Ph.D.

Selected Titles in the Series:
Clinical Methods and Practicum in Speech-Language Pathology by M. N. Hegde, Ph.D.,
    and Deborah Davis, M.A.
Applied Phonetics: The Sounds of American English by Harold T. Edwards, Ph.D.
The Acoustic Analysis of Speech by Raymond D. Kent, Ph.D., and Charles Read, Ph.D.
Introduction to Sound: Acoustics for the Hearing and Speech Sciences by Charles E. Speaks, Ph.D.
Assessment in Speech-Language Pathology: A Resource Manual by Kenneth G. Shipley, Ph.D.,
    and Julie G. McAfee, M.A.
Clinical Speech and Voice Measurement : Laboratory Exercises by Robert F. Orlikoff, Ph.D.,
    and Ronald J. Baken, Ph.D.
 Optimizing Theories and Experiments by Randall C. Robey, Ph.D., and Martin C. Schultz, Ph.D.

Also available:

A Singular Manual of Textbook Preparation by M. N. Hegde, Ph.D.

Published by Singular Publishing Group, Inc.
4284 41st Street
San Diego, CA 92105-1197

© 1994 by M. N. Hegde

Printed in the United States of America by McNaughton & Gunn
Typeset in 11 point Times New Roman

Library of Congress Cataloging-in-Publication Data

Hegde, M. N. (Mahabalagiri N.). 1941-
        A coursebook on scientific and professional writing in speech-language pathology /
    M. N. Hegde
            p.   cm. — (Singular Textbook Series)
        Includes biobliographic references
        ISBN 1-56593-260-9
            1. Speech disorders—Authorship—Handbooks, manuals, etc.
    2. Language disorders—Authorship—Handbooks, manuals, etc.
    3. Medical Writing—Handbooks, manuals, etc.   I. Title.
    II. Series.
        {DNLM: 1. Writing. 2. Speech-Language Pathology—education.   WZ
    345 H462s 1994}
    808', 06661-dc20
    DLM/DLC
    for Library of Congress

93-5286
CIP

BRIEF TABLE OF CONTENTS

See Pages 363-367 for Detailed Table of Contents

PREFACE

Teaching and learning to write in a technical and professional language is an important part of education in speech-language pathology. However, students often do not begin to acquire acceptable writing skills until they enroll in clinical practicum or in graduate research seminars in which professional and scientific writing are required. But many students are not adequately prepared for such writing.

Students who have taken courses on writing offered in other departments still do not have adequate technical and professional writing skills. To write well, students need to write and receive specific feedback. Students should rewrite and have multiple opportunities to practice the same type of skills and receive feedback every step of the way.

There are many books on writing, but few that give opportunities to practice writing as the examples are given. Most instructors know that simply asking students to read various books on good writing does not generate writing skills. Also, most writing courses are designed to teach rules of grammar, not writing. However, a good writer need not recite rules of grammar. Therefore, I have designed this new type of book which I call a *coursebook*. I have used this book in teaching technical and professional writing skills to undergraduate students with good results. This book makes it possible not only to show and tell what acceptable writing is but also to have students practice such writing immediately, on the facing pages of the same book.

I hope that instructors of courses on writing, research methods and graduate seminars, and clinical supervisors will find this book helpful in teaching technical and professional writing skills to students. In the *Introduction,* I have described the different methods of using this book. I welcome comments and suggestions from students and instructors who use this book.

INTRODUCTION

WHAT IS A *COURSEBOOK?*

A *coursebook* is a new type of book. It is a book that students not only read, but write on as well. It includes features of a textbook, a book of exercises, a resource manual, a laboratory manual, and an instructor's manual or handbook. By combining elements of different types of teaching tools, a coursebook becomes a unique and practical teaching tool.

The most important aspect of this coursebook is the way the left-hand and right-hand pages are designed. Most left-hand pages show specific examples of general, scientific, or professional writing. In many cases, both the incorrect and correct versions are shown. The corresponding right-hand pages require the student to write correctly. Typically, the facing pages contain the same rules or exemplars; one to read about, and the other to write on.

Different forms of coursebooks may be designed. My coursebook on *Aphasia and other Neurogenic Language Disorders* (Singular Publishing Group, 1994) illustrates a different kind of coursebook though both share a common feature: students read them as well as write on them. This coursebook is designed to generate good writing skills in students in speech-language pathology. The learning and teaching of writing skills can be frustrating to both the student and the instructor. Instructors know that merely extolling good writing and asking students to read some of the many available books on how to write well are not effective. Teaching writing skills is time- and effort-intensive because unless students have examples to follow and feedback to use, their skills do not improve. Students have to write, receive feedback, and rewrite. While it does not obviate the need for writing and rewriting, this coursebook makes that task somewhat more practical for both the student and the instructor.

This coursebook is designed with the following assumptions:

- It is not necessary to have students memorize the rules of grammar to write well
- Students should have many examples of the skills they are expected to learn
- Students should read an exemplar and write one immediately
- Students should write multiple exemplars
- Given exemplars and the student writing should go hand-in-hand
- To the extent possible, students should receive feedback in the classroom itself

HOW THIS COURSEBOOK MAY BE USED

This book has three parts. Part A is designed to teach some basic writing skills that are a foundation for any type of good writing. Part B is designed to teach scientific writing, mostly according to the third edition of the *Publication Manual of the American Psychological Association* (1983). Part C helps teach professional writing, including assessment reports, treatment plans, progress reports, and professional correspondence.

Both clinical supervisors and academic course instructors may use this book to teach scientific and professional writing skills. The book may be used in the following contexts:

- A course on writing
- Courses on research methods and introduction to graduate studies
- Clinical practica and internships
- Independent studies in writing skills
- Informally assigned work to help individual students master good writing skills

A course taught over a semester or quarter offers the most effective context to use this book. However, students enrolled in clinical practicum and courses on research methods will find many opportunities to practice technical and professional writing skills in the book. Also, the book is written in such a way as to help implement independent studies and informal writing assignments that are designed to remediate student-specific deficiencies in writing. The book or parts of the book may be assigned to students who complete the writing assignments shown on the right-hand pages. Multiple exemplars and boxed prompts on the right-hand pages reduce mistakes.

GIVING FEEDBACK TO STUDENTS

Through multiple exemplars and assignments, the book itself gives feedback to the student. Still, the instructor should give as much feedback as possible. A problem instructors face is to find time to read large amounts of writing from a big class and give student-specific feedback. This problem may be overcome by having the students complete the writing assignments on the right-hand pages before they come to class. In each class period, all students read aloud at least some portions of their writing. The instructor then gives immediate verbal feedback and all students make corrections on their writing. The instructor makes sure that every student reads some portion of his or her writing and that all students take the feedback seriously. When this method is used the instructor may read only the tests given to the students.

Nonetheless, the instructor will have given student-specific feedback on writing. In this method, the instructor spends most, if not all of the time in class periods on giving feedback to students on their writing. This contrasts with the traditional method of teaching writing in which most of the time is spent on lecturing about rules of writing. It is hoped that this coursebook method of teaching will facilitate more writing from students and more feedback from instructors while still keeping both to a manageable level.

HOW THIS BOOK WAS PREPARED AND PRODUCED

This book was prepared and produced entirely on a computer word processor. The looks and the format of a computer-printed document is retained purposefully to give the student a sense of writing with a word processor. Without right justification and some acceptable variation in style and format, the book is thought to reflect how most professionals write. For these reasons, the look of a formally typeset book is avoided.

PART A

FOUNDATIONS OF SCIENTIFIC

AND

PROFESSIONAL WRITING

A.1. BASIC RULES OF USAGE

A.1.1. DO NOT TURN A PLURAL INTO A POSSESSIVE

(Do not use an unnecessary apostrophe.)

Incorrect	Correct	Note
The characteristic's of aphasia are well known.	The characteristics of aphasia are well known.	
The characteristics' of aphasia are well known.		
In the 1970's, the clinicians began to treat language disorders.	In the 1970s the clinicians began to treat language disorders.	A common mistake.

A.1.2. DO NOT TURN A POSSESSIVE INTO A PLURAL

(Use anapostrophe when needed.)

Incorrect	Correct	Note
The patients resistance to treatment was high.	The patient's resistance to treatment was high.	Singular possessives
The clients prognosis is good.	The client's prognosis is good.	
The clinicians motivation to treat is an important variable.	The clinicians' motivation to treat is an important variable.	Plural possessive

A.1. BASIC RULES OF USAGE

A.1.1. DO NOT TURN A PLURAL INTO A POSSESSIVE

(Do not use an unnecessary apostrophe.)

Incorrect	Write Correctly
Dysarthric patients' will have a history of neurologic involvement.	
Many factors' affect the treatment outcome.	
The problems of the 80's will persist into the 90's	

A.1.2. DO NOT TURN A POSSESSIVE INTO A PLURAL

(Use an apostrophe when needed.)

Incorrect	Write Correctly
I will train the clients mother in response maintenance.	
Poorly drawn stimulus pictures can reduce a treatments effectiveness.	
The treatment settings influence cannot be ignored. *Hint: The sentence contains a plural possessive.*	

A.1.3. USE A SERIAL COMMA

The comma after *blue* and before *and* in *Red, blue, and green* is called a serial comma. When you use three or more terms connected with a single conjunction, use a comma after each except the last term which follows the conjunction.

Incorrect	Correct	Note
The child had multiple misarticulations, language delay and a hearing loss.	The child had multiple misarticulations, language delay, and a hearing loss.	The use of conjunction *and*
Our clinicians are intelligent, compassionate and competent.	Our clinicians are intelligent, compassionate, and competent.	
Each token may be exchanged for a sticker, piece of gum or a small toy.	Each token may be exchanged for a sticker, a piece of gum, or a small toy.	The use of conjunction *or*

A.1.4. DO NOT USE A SERIAL COMMA WHEN YOU WRITE ONLY TWO PARALLEL TERMS AND CONNECT THEM WITH A CONJUNCTION

Incorrect	Correct	Note
The patient with aphasia had naming, and comprehension problems.	The patient with aphasia had naming and comprehension problems.	In each case, only two terms are joined by a different conjunction (*and, or*)
Plastic tokens, or stickers will be used as reinforcers.	Plastic tokens or stickers will be used as reinforcers.	

A.1.3. USE A SERIAL COMMA

Incorrect	Write Correctly
The training targets will be the correct production of the plural morpheme, the auxiliary and the copula.	
Correct responses will be reinforced with verbal praise, smile or tokens.	
Sensori, neural and sensorineural hearing losses must be distinguished.	

A.1.4. DO NOT USE A SERIAL COMMA WHEN YOU WRITE ONLY TWO PARALLEL TERMS AND CONNECT THEM WITH A CONJUNCTION

Incorrect	Write Correctly
The child exhibited omissions, and distortions of several speech sounds.	
The treatment may be started at the word, or the phrase level.	
Aural rehabilitation begins with the selection of an analog, or digital hearing aid.	

A.1.5. USE A COMMA TO SEPARATE PARENTHETIC EXPRESSIONS WHEN YOU DO NOT USE PARENTHESES

Incorrect	Correct
The woman who stuttered though she could not remember it had received treatment before.	The woman who stuttered, though she could not remember it, had received treatment before.
The client who was extremely dysfluent hesitated before starting to read aloud.	The client, who was extremely dysfluent, hesitated before starting to read aloud.

A.1.6. PLACE A COMMA BEFORE A CONJUNCTION INTRODUCING AN INDEPENDENT CLAUSE

Incorrect	Correct
The clinician suggested a treatment program but the client was unresponsive.	The clinician suggested a treatment program, but the patient was unresponsive.
The man was diagnosed with aphasia and the prognosis for recovery was poor.	The man was diagnosed with aphasia, and the prognosis for recovery was poor.

A.1.7. DO NOT JOIN INDEPENDENT CLAUSES WITH A COMMA WHEN THE CLAUSES ARE NOT JOINED BY A CONJUNCTION

Join them with a semicolon.
You can rewrite the two independent clauses as two separate sentences, however.

Incorrect	Correct
Stuttering is a speech problem, it should not be ignored.	Stuttering is a speech problem; it should not be ignored.
	Stuttering is a speech disorder. It should not be ignored.

A.1.5. USE A COMMA TO SEPARATE PARENTHETIC EXPRESSIONS WHEN YOU DO NOT USE PARENTHESES

Incorrect	Write Correctly
The child with misarticulations though socially competent was not doing well in the school.	
The client who had a severe form of aphasia could not readily respond when asked to name objects.	

A.1.6. PLACE A COMMA BEFORE A CONJUNCTION INTRODUCING AN INDEPENDENT CLAUSE

Incorrect	Write Correctly
The client's mother was asked to attend all treatment sessions but her attendance was poor.	
The father conducted treatment sessions at home and the progress was excellent.	

A.1.7. DO NOT JOIN INDEPENDENT CLAUSES WITH A COMMA WHEN THE CLAUSES ARE NOT JOINED BY A CONJUNCTION

Incorrect	Write Correctly
Dementia is a neurologically based language disorder, it often is undetected in many nursing homes.	1. 2.
Early treatment of stuttering is effective, this is unknown to some clinicians.	1. 2.

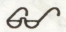

A.1.8. USE A DASH TO SET OFF AN ABRUPT BREAK OR INTERRUPTION

Note: Typesetters and manuals of advanced word processors call it the *em dash*. With most word processors, you use a special code to type an *em dash*, not the dash on the keyboard.

Incorrect	Correct
The speech discrimination test, a standard portion of any audiological diagnostic evaluation revealed no significant problem.	The speech discrimination test—a standard procedure of any audiological diagnostic evaluation—revealed no significant problems.
The administration of a pure probe, if it is administered at all requires much prior work.	The administration of a pure probe—if it is administered at all—requires much prior work.

Note: There is no space separating the *em dash* and the word that precedes or follows it.

A.1.9. AGREEMENT

Subject and verb should agree in number.
The terms that intervene between the noun phrase and the verb do not affect agreement.

Incorrect	Correct	Note
No single dysfluency type—prolongations, interjections, or word repetitions—justify diagnosis.	No single dysfluency type—prolongations, interjections, or word repetitions—justifies diagnosis.	No single dysfluency *type justifies* diagnosis.
She is one of the clinicians who is always prepared for her sessions.	She is one of the clinicians who are always prepared for their sessions.	*clinicians* who *are*
For many reasons, the stuttering person believes that they cannot be treated.	For many reasons, the stuttering person believes that he or she cannot be treated. *or* For many reasons, stuttering persons believe that they cannot be treated.	stuttering person *believes* that *he or she*
These techniques, when used appropriately by a competent clinician, is known to be effective.	These techniques, when used appropriately by a competent clinician, are known to be effective.	*techniques are* known to

A.1.8. USE A DASH TO SET OFF AN ABRUPT BREAK OR INTERRUPTION

Incorrect	Write Correctly
Modeling the target response, a basic procedure in language treatment, will be used whenever the client does not imitate.	
Treatment of stuttering, unless the clinician is an ardent believer in spontaneous recovery, should be started as early as possible.	
The incidence of noise-induced hearing loss, a hazardous but controllable by-product of civilization, is on the increase.	

A.1.9. AGREEMENT

Incorrect	Write Correctly
A disorder of articulation—whether it contains a few or many misarticulations—indicate a need for treatment.	
He is one of those individuals who is always late.	
A client who thinks that the clinician should do everything may not take responsibility for their progress.	
Tokens, when dispensed immediately for a correct response, increases the rate of progress.	

Agreement (continued)

Incorrect	Correct	Note
Error scores, along with the correct score, was used in the analysis.	Error scores, along with the correct score, were used in the analysis.	Error *scores were* used
Every child and adult go through the same procedure.	Every child and adult goes through the same procedure.	A singular verb is used when *each* or *every* precedes a compound subject joined by *and*.
Either verbal praise or informative feedback are combined with modeling.	Either verbal praise or informative feedback is combined with modeling.	When two subjects are linked by *or*, *either/or*, or *neither/nor*, the verb must be plural if both the subjects are plural and singular if both the subjects are singular. In this case, both are singular.
Neither the stimuli nor the response consequences was well planned.	Neither the stimuli nor the response consequences were well planned.	In this case, both are plural.
Neither the treatments nor the result are replicable.	Neither the treatments nor the result is replicable.	When a singular and a plural subject are linked by *neither/nor*, *either/or*, or *not only/but also*, the verb form is determined by the subject that is nearer to it. As in *result is...* *settings, tend to...*
Not only the treatment procedure, but also the treatment settings, tends to have an effect on the client's progress.	Not only the treatment procedure, but also the treatment settings, tend to have an effect on the client's progress	
Mother and child was interviewed together.	Mother and child were interviewed together.	Compound subjects joined by *and* have plural verbs.
Who says "country and western" are dead?	Who says "country and western" is dead?	Expressions containing *and* that suggest a single concept use singular verbs. *Country and western* is a single concept, though joined by *and*.
Both of us is busy.	Both of us are busy.	A few indefinite pronouns (*both, many, several, few, others*) are always plural and take plural verbs.
Either of them are acceptable.	Either of them is acceptable.	Most other indefinite pronouns (*another, anyone, everyone, each, either, neither, anything, everything, something,* and *somebody*) are singular and take singular verbs.

Agreement (continued)

Incorrect	Write Correctly
Percent dysfluency rates, along with the frequency of each dysfluency, is presented in Table 1.	
Every client and the selected family member receive training in recognizing the target response.	
Either time-out or response cost for incorrect responses are combined with positive reinforcement for correct responses.	
Neither the procedures nor the outcome are clearly described.	
Either verbal feedback or tokens is given to the client for her correct responses.	
The clinician and the client's sister was in the same treatment room.	
Who says "rock 'n' roll are for the devils?"	
Several of the group is unhappy.	
Either of the two techniques are effective.	
Some of this mess are your responsibility.	
Some of the effects is unexplained.	
None of the children is improving with this procedure.	
None of the effect are due to treatment.	
The twin pair were tested in a single session.	
The majority do not agree.	
Politics are full of scoundrels	

Agreement (continued)

Incorrect	Correct	Take Note
Some of this effect are understandable.	Some of this effect is understandable.	Some indefinite pronouns (*some, all, none, any, more,* and *most*) can be singular or plural. The verb form is singular or plural depending upon the noun the pronoun refers to.
The group were tested in a single session.	The group was tested in a single session.	Collective nouns can take singular verbs (if they refer to a single unit) or plural verbs (if they refer to individuals or elements of that unit.)
The majority were against the idea. A majority of people was against the idea.	The majority was against the idea. A majority of people were against the idea.	*The majority* is singular; *a majority of people* is plural.
The news are bad.	The news is bad.	
Statistics are an exciting field.	Statistics is an exciting field.	Some words that are typically in the plural form still take singular verbs.
Economics are not an exact science.	Economics is not an exact science.	
Statistics shows that the prevalence of phonological disorders in the preschool children is high.	*Statistics show* that the prevalence of phonological disorders in the preschool children is high.	When the word *statistics refers not to the subject but to some numbers, it takes the plural.*

Agreement (continued)

Incorrect	Write Correctly
The subjects in the group was tested once.	
The majority were unimpressed.	
A majority of clinicians tends to use this procedure.	
Statistics are not an easy subject.	
Some of her statistics was interesting.	

A.1.10. USE MODIFIERS CORRECTLY

To avoid confusion in the use of modifiers, keep the related words together. This is pointed out in the third column.

Incorrect	Correct	Note
The author and her assistants tested the hearing of all subjects using the procedure described earlier.	The author and her assistants, using the procedure described earlier, tested the hearing of all subjects.	Who used the procedure? Not the subjects!
Distant and mysterious, he stared at the sky.	He stared at the distant and mysterious sky.	Who was mysterious and distant? Not he!
Several additional effects are observed using this technique in clients.	Several additional effects are observed in clients using this technique.	Who observed effects in whom?
Using the standard procedure, the subjects were screened for hearing problems by the experimenter.	Using the standard procedure, the experimenter screened the subjects for hearing problems.	Who used the standard procedure?
The study *merely* provided a partial support for the hypothesis. Establishing the target behaviors in the clinic without concern for maintenance is hardly sufficient.	The study provided *merely* a partial support for the hypothesis. It is hardly sufficient to establish the target behaviors in the clinic without concern for maintenance.	Place the following modifiers immediately before the words they modify: *almost, only, even, hardly, merely, nearly, exactly, scarcely, just,* and *simply*

A.1.11. DO NOT USE PRONOUNS WHOSE REFERENTS ARE NOT CLEAR

Incorrect	Correct	Note
I will use toys and pictures as stimuli, and give reinforcers for correct responses. *They* will be employed only when the response rate does not increase.	I will use toys and pictures as stimuli and give reinforcers for correct responses. *These reinforcers* will be employed only when the response rate does not increase.	*They* refers to what? Correct responses or reinforcers?
A lesion in Broca's area in the left frontal cortex causes Broca's aphasia. *It* may be diagnosed only after careful examination.	A lesion in Broca's aphasia, in the left frontal cortex, may be diagnosed only after careful examination. Such a lesion causes Broca's aphasia.	What may be diagnosed? The corrected statement says it is the lesion.

A.1.10. USE MODIFIERS CORRECTLY

Incorrect	Write Correctly
The clinician treated stuttering persons using the syllable stretching procedure.	
Consistent with other studies, Smith and Smith (1993) found that cochlear implants are beneficial. Hint: what were consistent? Results or the authors?	
The treatment only was partially effective.	
Using the Utah Test, the children's language was screened by the experimenter.	

A.1.11. DO NOT USE PRONOUNS WHOSE REFERENTS ARE NOT CLEAR

Incorrect	Write Correctly
The treatment procedure will include various stimuli, modeling, and positive feedback. *It* will be used only when the child does not imitate, however. (*It* refers to what?)	
The results of many studies, conducted by several investigators have confirmed this. They indicate that we should program maintenance. (*They* refer to what?)	

A.1.12. DO NOT BREAK A SENTENCE INTO TWO

Incorrect	Correct
Upon subjective evaluation. The client's voice was judged normal.	Upon subjective evaluation, the client's voice was judged normal.
The client finally agreed to be tested. After much coaxing from his wife.	After much coaxing from his wife, the client finally agreed to be tested.
I work with 10 children. All with a severe articulation problem.	I work with 10 children, all with a severe articulation problem.
Many hearing impaired children have delayed oral language. And also may have voice problems.	Many hearing impaired children have delayed oral language and also may have voice problems.

A.1.13. DO NOT TURN AN ADJECTIVE INTO A NOUN

Incorrect	Correct	Note
The *paraplegic* also has aphasia.	The patient with paraplegia also has aphasia.	
The *aphasic* has naming problems.	The person with aphasia has naming problems.	The incorrect versions put the disability first, not the person.
The *autistic* has echolalia.	The child with autism has echolalia.	

A.1.14. DO NOT TURN A NOUN INTO A VERB

Incorrect	Correct	Note
We will *agendize* this matter for the next meeting.	We will place this matter on the next meeting's agenda.	The popular tendency to *ize* a noun has created many awkward verbs.
The treatment targets will be *prioritized*.	I will make a priority list of treatment targets.	
I *gifted* that to her.	I gave that to her as a gift.	
First, I *baselined* the target behaviors.	First, I established baselines of the target behaviors.	
The stuttering person was *therapized* by many clinicians.	1. The stuttering person had received therapy from many clinicians. 2. Many clinicians had treated the stuttering person.	

A.1.12. DO NOT BREAK A SENTENCE INTO TWO

Incorrect	Write Correctly
I will treat 12 children with language disorders. Divided into two groups.	
The child finally began to cooperate. After two sessions of crying.	
I tested the hearing of selected subjects. In a sound-treated room.	
The client made excellent progress. In the final four sessions.	

A.1.13. DO NOT TURN AN ADJECTIVE INTO A NOUN

Incorrect	Write Correctly
The dysarthric has multiple communicative disorders.	
The retarded's language is delayed.	
The hemiplegic has motor speech disorders.	

A.1.14. DO NOT TURN A NOUN INTO A VERB

Incorrect	Write Correctly
She hosted a dinner party.	
He guested on a TV show.	

A.1.15. USE THE PROPER CASE OF PRONOUN

Incorrect	Correct	Note
Between you and I	Between you and me.	
They have invited you and myself.	They have invited you and me.	
Her's is the big house.	Hers is the big house.	Possessive pronouns *hers*, *theirs*, *ours*, and *its* do not take the apostrophe.
It's tail is too bushy.	Its tail is too bushy.	
Its an effective procedure.	It's an effective procedure.	In formal writing, do not use this contracted form of *it is*.

A.1.16. A PARTICIPIAL PHRASE AT THE BEGINNING OF A SENTENCE MUST REFER TO THE GRAMMATICAL SUBJECT

Incorrect	Correct
On discussing treatment options with the client's family, *they* responded favorably to the clinician.	On discussing treatment options with the client's family, *the clinician* received favorable responses.
A clinician of great reputation, *I* asked her to treat the client.	A clinician of great reputation, *she* was asked to treat the client.

A.1.15. USE THE PROPER CASE OF PRONOUN

Incorrect	Write Correctly
You and myself should complete the assessment.	
He told Tom and I to finish the job.	
Their's is the clinic that specializes in myofunctional therapy.	
Its a convenient test to administer.	

A.1.16. A PARTICIPIAL PHRASE AT THE BEGINNING OF A SENTENCE MUST REFER TO THE GRAMMATICAL SUBJECT

Incorrect	Write Correctly
Inexperienced in the treatment of dysphagia, the treatment goals were thought to be easy to establish.	
Without a friend to study with, the failure was inevitable.	

A.2. BASIC RULES OF COMPOSITION

A.2.1. DESIGN A BROAD OUTLINE OF YOUR PAPER

Before you begin to write a paper, an essay, a report, or a book chapter, make a broad outline of it. In making an outline, think of what major topics you want to address in the paper. Study the following example.

Note that the author made some brief notes under each of the major topics to be addressed:

Theories of Language Acquisition

Bridgette Lopez

Brief historical introduction to the study of language

> *(the study of language is age-old, philosophers have studied it, many disciplines study it, and so forth.)*

Linguistic theories of language acquisition

> *(Descriptive linguistics, transformational generative grammar, semantic explanations, and so forth)*

Psychological theories of language acquisition

> *(Behavioral explanations, cognitive explanations, interactive explanations)*

Recent developments in theoretical explanations

> *(Attempts at integrating different views, suggestions from cross-cultural studies)*

Critical evaluation of theories

> *(lack of experimental support for most theories]*

Summary and conclusions

> *(Need for additional research; future directions)*

Note: There is no one correct outline for a topic. The first outline usually is modified.

A.2. BASIC RULES OF COMPOSITION

A.2.1. DESIGN A BROAD OUTLINE OF YOUR PAPER

Select a major academic or clinical topic and design an outline for it.
Show your notes.

A.2.2. DESIGN HEADINGS AND SUBHEADINGS OF YOUR PAPER

Use the headings and subheadings of your outline.
Think of additional headings and subheadings.
Give technical headings.
Prefer the shorter to the longer headings.
Try to have the same number of subheadings under major headings.
Use these headings in your paper.

Theories of Language Acquisition
Bridgette Lopez

Brief historical introduction to the study of language (Untitled)

Linguistic theories of language acquisition

   Descriptive Linguistic Theories
   Transformational Generative Theories
   Generative Semantic Theories
   Government and Binding Theory
   Recent Linguistic Developments

Psychological theories of language acquisition

   Behavioral Theories
   Cognitive Theories
   Interactional Theories

Recent developments in theoretical explanations

   Attempts at Integrating Different Views
   Suggestions from Cross-cultural Studies

Critical evaluation of theories

   Comparative Evaluation of Evidence
   Suggestions for Future Research

Summary and conclusions

References

Note: The example contains only two levels of heading. Additional levels of headings may be necessary for most papers.

A.2.2. DESIGN HEADINGS AND SUBHEADINGS OF YOUR PAPER

For the outline you have prepared under A.2.1., design headings and subheadings.

Revise your headings and subheadings until you can begin writing.

A.2.3. WRITE PARAGRAPHS THAT EXPRESS RELATED IDEAS

A paragraph expresses *related* ideas.
Different kinds of information should not be mixed-up in a paragraph.
Each paragraph should be a conceptual unit.

Incorrect	Correct	Note

The subjects will be 25 hearing impaired children. They will come from middle-class families. The children will be selected from a single school within the local school district. The parents of the children will have normal hearing. The intelligence of the children will be within normal limits. The selected subjects will not have any other physical or psychological disability.
 	
    The children will be selected from a single school within the local school district.
	The subjects will be 25 hearing impaired children. They will come from middle-class families. ~~The children will be selected from a single school within the local school district~~. The parents of the children will have normal hearing. The intelligence of the children will be within normal limits. The selected subjects will not have any other physical or psychological disability.
	
	    The children will be selected from a single school within the local school district.
		The first paragraph describes the subject characteristics. The stricken sentence introduces a different idea (that of subject selection). This should be told in a separate paragraph.

The client will be seen two times a week in 30-minute sessions. The initial target behaviors will be the correct production of five phonemes. In the beginning, the client will be trained on discrete trials. Later, conversational speech will be used to train the target phonemes.
 	
    The initial training procedure will include discrete trials. A picture will be used to evoke the target phoneme in words.
	The client will be seen two times a week in 30-minute sessions. The initial target behaviors will be the correct production of five phonemes. ~~In the beginning, the client will be trained on discrete trials. Later, conversational speech will be used to train the target phonemes.~~
	
	    The initial training procedure will include discrete trials. A picture will be used to evoke the target phoneme in words.
	
	    In the final stage of treatment, conversational speech will be used to stabilize the production of target phonemes.
		This paragraph is about target behaviors, not treatment procedures. The stricken sentences are intrusive in that they introduce a different topic. This paragraph is about the training procedure.
		
		A separate paragraph is necessary to describe the final stage of treatment.

A.2.3. WRITE PARAGRAPHS THAT EXPRESS RELATED IDEAS

Incorrect	Write Correctly
Mr. Samsungson reported that he began to notice hearing problems some five months ago. His wife agreed that it was about that time that her husband began to turn up the volume of their television. He has been in good physical health. He also began to complain that his wife mumbles her speech. Until about five months ago, Mr. Samsungson had no physical or sensory complaints.	

Write a Mixed-up Paragraph	Rewrite It Correctly

A.2.4. DO NOT WRITE PARAGRAPHS THAT ARE TOO LONG

Break longer paragraphs into shorter ones.

Too Long	About Right	Note
Assessment of Timmy's speech and language behaviors will include an orofacial examination, a hearing screening, and administration of the Thompson Vocabulary Test, the Jenson Test of Articulatory Performance, the Conduction Test of Central Auditory Processing, the Tinson Test of Developmental Dysarthria, and the Shanks Test of Syntactic Constructions. In addition, an extended conversational speech sample will be recorded. A second conversational speech sample will be recorded in the clinic after a one-week interval. Finally, the parents will be asked to bring two 10-minute samples of audio taped conversational speech from home. The results of this assessment will be integrated with information obtained through case history, reports from other specialists, and information gathered through interview of Timmy's parents. The client's performance on the selected standardized tests will be analyzed according to the test manuals. The conversational speech samples will be analyzed to determine the accuracy of phoneme productions and language structures. The number of phonemes correctly produced, the number of syntactic structures correctly used, and the number of pragmatic rules appropriately followed also will be determined. Besides, the mean length of utterance will be calculated using the Brown method. A general measure of pragmatic use of language also will be evaluated from the observations.	Assessment of Timmy's speech and language behaviors will include an orofacial examination, a hearing screening, and administration of the Thompson Vocabulary Test, the Jenson Test of Articulatory Performance, the Conduction Test of Central Auditory Processing, the Tinson Test of Developmental Dysarthria, and the Shanks Test of Syntactic Constructions. In addition, an extended conversational speech sample will be recorded. A second conversational speech sample will be recorded in the clinic after a one-week interval. Finally, the parents will be asked to bring two 10-minute samples of audio taped conversational speech from home. The results of this assessment will be integrated with information obtained through case history, reports from other specialists, and information gathered through interview of Timmy's parents. The client's performance on the selected standardized tests will be analyzed according to the test manuals. The conversational speech samples will be analyzed to determine the accuracy of phoneme productions and language structures. The number of phonemes correctly produced, the number of syntactic structures correctly used, and the number of pragmatic rules appropriately followed also will be determined. Besides, the mean length of utterance will be calculated using the Brown method. A general measure of pragmatic use of language also will be evaluated from the observations.	The long paragraph has been broken into smaller ones, each describing a set of related ideas.

A.2.4. DO NOT WRITE PARAGRAPHS THAT ARE TOO LONG

Too Long	Rewrite To Make It About Right
Aural rehabilitation is an extended process in which a hearing impaired person is helped to make use of his or her residual hearing. The process begins with hearing testing, but it does not end with it. The process does not end even with a prescription for, or fitting of, a hearing aid. The purchase of a hearing aid is the beginning of aural rehabilitation. The patient should be first familiarized with the workings of the hearing aid. The patient should learn to change the battery, turn on the aid, adjust the volume, and so forth. The patient should know how to take care of the aid, clean it periodically, and protect it from shock and other hazards. The patient also should know when to take it for service. But even more importantly, the patient should know how to benefit from the aid. Initially, the hearing aid's amplification of sound and noise may irritate the person or cause discomfort. Some patients may get headaches until they get used to the aid's amplified sound. The patient should know how to handle the incoming, amplified signal. The audiologist should teach the client to recognize the meaning of sound the patient can now hear.	

A.2.5. DO NOT WRITE ONE-SENTENCE PARAGRAPHS

To create an effect on the reader, you can occasionally break this rule in popular writing, but in scientific and professional writing, avoid one-sentence paragraphs.

Inappropriate	Appropriate	Note
The client's correct production of the target phonemes began to increase in the fourth treatment session. During the sixth session, the correct response rate increased from a baseline rate of 27 to 78% . Then the reinforcement schedule was changed from continuous to an FR4. The client continued to make progress.	The client's correct production of the target phonemes began to increase in the fourth treatment session. During the sixth session, the correct response rate increased from a baseline rate of 27 to 78%. Though the reinforcement schedule was then changed from continuous to an FR4, the client continued to make progress.	The one-sentence paragraph stands alone with nothing to connect to. Note that when the two paragraphs are combined, some change in the wording may be necessary to provide transition.

A.2.5. DO NOT WRITE ONE-SENTENCE PARAGRAPHS

Write Four Paragraphs, Each With a Single Sentence	Integrate the Four Into a Single Paragraph

A.2.6. BEGIN AND END MOST PARAGRAPHS WITH TRANSITORY SENTENCES

Lack of transition breaks the flow of thought and confuses the reader.
To achieve smooth transition, **do**:

    end and begin adjacent paragraphs with a related idea.
    suggest what will be said in the next paragraph.
    make reference to what was said in the previous paragraph.

However, **do not**:

    introduce new topics abruptly.
    randomly shift topics across paragraphs.

Rough Transition	Smoother Transition	Note
1. Methods of analysis of articulatory errors have undergone many changes. Traditionally, the clinicians have made the sound-by-sound analysis to judge the accuracy of individual sound productions. 2. In the place-voice-manner analysis, sounds are classified into patterns based on these phonetic features. Errors also are similarly classified. 3. Phonological processes are simplifications of speech sound productions that help classify multiple errors into groups or patterns. Another approach is that of distinctive feature analysis, which was suggested before the phonological process approach.	1. Methods of analysis of articulatory errors have undergone many changes. Traditionally, the clinicians have made the sound-by-sound analysis to judge the acuracy of individual sound productions. Therefore, *there is no attempt to see a pattern in the errors* based on an underlying principle. 2. The first approach to see a *pattern in the errors* was based on the place-voice-manner analysis. In this approach, sounds are classified into patterns based on the three phonetic features. Therefore, errors also are similarly classified. This classification resulted in somewhat *simplified patterns of errors.* 3. A method of classification resulting in more *complex patterns of errors* was suggested by the next approach: analysis of the distinctive features of speech sounds. Soon, however, a new approach based on *phonological theories* was proposed. 4. *Phonological theories* proposed that phonological processes, which are patterned simplifications of speech sound productions, explain errors of articulation. These processes help classify multiple errors into groups or patterns.	The first paragraph of the first column set the stage for a historical view. But with no transition and no historical sense, the second paragraph is isolated. The first two paragraphs of the second column are related because of the common, italicized words. A theme flows from the first to the second paragraph. The third paragraph of the first column abruptly introduces the phonological process approach. The rewriting achieves smoother transition as shown by a repeated theme (italicized words in the second and the third paragraphs). The third paragraph in the first column confuses the historical sequence because of an abrupt shift to phonological approach before mentioning the distinctive feature approach.

A.2.6. BEGIN AND END MOST PARAGRAPHS WITH TRANSITORY SENTENCES

Rough Transition	Rewrite With Smoother Transition
The treatment targets for this client (with aphasia) will include naming five common objects: *cup, book, shirt, sock,* and *shoe*. The baseline data show that the client can name them only with 5% accuracy within 20 sec of stimulus presentation. These naming responses were selected for training because of their obvious usefulness to the client. The training sessions will last 50 min. The training will start at the word level. Eventually, the names will be integrated into phrases and conversational speech. The client will be seen two times a week. Modeling and reinforcement will be used in training. Pictures of the selected objects will be used in training sessions. Each stimulus will be presented on discrete trials. The clinician will place a picture in front of the client and ask "What is this?" Immediately, the clinician will model the label for the client to imitate. If the client does not imitate within 10 sec, the stimulus will be withdrawn and another presented. If the client responds correctly, verbal praise will be presented. If the client does not respond within 10 sec of modeling, the clinician will not say anything. The clinician will move on to the next trial with a different picture. When the client correctly imitates the label on five consecutive trials, modeling will be withdrawn. If necessary, modeling will be faded. If the client does not respond when the modeling is withdrawn, modeling will be reinstated. Modeling will then be faded. When the client correctly labels an object on 10 consecutive evoked trails, the clinician will shift training to the phrase level.	

Hint: Different kinds of information are mixed-up in different paragraphs and there is little transition between paragraphs. Examine each sentence to see if it belongs in the paragraph. Write transitory sentences at the end and the beginning of paragraphs.

A.2.7. USE THE ACTIVE VOICE

Passive sentences are long and indirect. In most cases, they can be avoided.

Passive	Preferred Active
The supervisor was the person with whom I spoke.	I spoke to the supervisor.
The children were brought to the clinic by their mothers.	The mothers brought their children to the clinic.
The target responses will be modeled by the clinician.	The clinician will model the target responses.
When the target behaviors are selected, stimulus materials will be prepared.	After selecting the target behaviors, I will prepare the stimulus materials.

A.2.8. PREFER SHORTER TO LONGER SENTENCES

Maintain some variety, however.
Alternate longer sentences with shorter ones.

Longer Sentences	Preferred Shorter Sentences	Note
Many clinicians who employ the traditional method of articulation training tend to use nonsense syllables in the early stages of training, along with an emphasis on ear training with a view to promote auditory discrimination of speech sounds.	Many clinicians employ the traditional method of articulation training. In this method, the clinicians use nonsense syllables in the early stages of training. The training emphasis is on the auditory discrimination of speech sounds.	One sentence has been broken into three. Shorter sentences are easier to read and understand.
The many compounding problems of the hearing impaired child include social isolation, academic difficulties, problems in language learning, and many others that when unchecked by a well designed management plan, can lead to additional problems later in life which are then very difficult to manage.	The many compounding problems of the hearing impaired child include social isolation, academic difficulties, and language learning problems. Unless checked by a well designed management plan, these problems can lead to additional difficulties later in life. Such long-standing problems are difficult to manage.	The maze of long sentences obscures a chain of ideas or events. The shorter sentences make them clearer to the reader. Some long sentences contain unnecessary words that can be cut out to shorten them.

A.2.7. USE THE ACTIVE VOICE

Passive	Rewrite In Preferred Active Terms
Central auditory processing problems may be assessed by various tests.	
The client's behavior problems were not controlled by the clinician.	
There are many procedures that may be used in aural rehabilitation.	
The clinician was upset by the child's noncooperative behavior.	

A.2.8. PREFER THE SHORTER TO THE LONGER SENTENCES

Longer Sentences	Rewrite in Shorter Sentences
Many clinicians, who believe that auditory training is an important part of aural rehabilitation of hearing impaired children, nonetheless do not appreciate the need for such training in case of adult hearing impaired individuals, though it is well established that the recognition and discrimination of speech sounds is an integral part of any program of aural rehabilitation designed for individuals of all ages.	
While the psychoanalytic theory has stated that stuttering is due primarily to oral and anal regression during infancy, the behavioral view has asserted that stuttering is due to faulty conditioning, and the neurophysiological theories have implicated either the auditory system with defective feedback loops, the laryngeal mechanism with improper neural control, or the brain with its problems in language processing.	

A.2.9. USE POSITIVE TERMS

Instead of saying what it is not, say what it is.

Negative	Preferred Positive
The client often did not come to the treatment sessions at the appointed time.	The client often came late to treatment sessions.
These treatment procedures are not very effective.	These treatment procedures are ineffective.
The results of our tests do not suggest that the client does not have central auditory processing problems.	The results of our tests suggest that the client has central auditory processing problems.
I do not believe that the client does not have a phonological disorder.	The client has a phonological disorder.
I do not think that these procedures will not work with aphasia.	I think that these procedures will work with aphasia. 2. These procedures will work with aphasia.
The man is not honest.	The man is dishonest.
The clinician did not pay any attention to the supervisor's suggestion.	The clinician ignored the supervisor's suggestion.

A.2.10. AVOID TOO MANY QUALIFICATIONS

Too many qualifications make your writing timid, weak, and uncertain. The reader will be unsure of what you say. Let your statements be as definite as the *observations warrant.*

Overly Qualified and Weak	Stronger and Clearer
It is possible that some clinicians do not have a very strong belief in the validity of this theory.	1. Some clinicians doubt the validity of this theory. 2. Some clinicians reject this theory.
The data may possibly suggest that in at least some cases, the technique may have some limited use.	The data suggest that the technique may be useful in some cases.
It would be beneficial to use this assessment procedure with children thought it may or may not be just as effective with adults.	This assessment procedure may be more useful with children than with adults.
It may be possible to use the criterion of 90% correct response rate before dismissing the client.	The dismissal criterion will be 90% correct response rate.

A.2.9. USE POSITIVE TERMS

Negative	Rewrite in Preferred Positive Terms
The instructor did not have much confidence in the student's explanation.	
The nativist theory does not do a great job of explaining language acquisition.	
Asking yes/no questions may not be an effective method of evoking continuous speech from a child.	
Some clinicians believe that phoneme auditory discrimination training may not be an efficient method of treatment.	
Surgical procedures may not be very effective in the rehabilitation of certain types of hearing impairment.	

A.2.10. AVOID TOO MANY QUALIFICATIONS

Overly Qualified and Weak	Stronger and Clearer
Theory may be of some value in explaining at least a small aspect of this complex phenomenon.	
I hope that with the help of this new procedure, I may be able to have some effect on the child's communication.	
Though I am not certain, I am favorably disposed to using the rate reduction procedure in the treatment of stuttering.	
I expect that I may be able to convince the parents that they may consider the possibility of holding informal treatment sessions at home.	
I expect that in all likelihood the digital hearing aid may prove to be beneficial for this client.	
Some data suggest that it is not entirely out of the realm of possibility that mild hearing loss may have some, even if minimum, effect on language acquisition in young children.	

A.2.11. USE DEFINITE, SPECIFIC, CONCRETE LANGUAGE

Avoid the overuse of generalized terms whose meanings are not clear.
Be specific in describing symptoms of disorders, behaviors, procedures,
effects, services, and so forth.

Incorrect	Correct
In all likelihood, the treatment seems to have had some positive effect on the life of the client.	Possibly, treatment helped the client speak more fluently.
Various visual and auditory stimulus input methods will be used in treatment.	Pictures, objects, action figures, and tape–recorded models of speech sound productions will be used in treatment.
I will make sure that the parents support Johnny's production of target behaviors at home.	I will ask the parents to praise Johnny at home for his correct production of speech sounds.
A variety of grammatic morphemes will be the treatment targets.	Many grammatic morphemes, including the regular plural, possessive, the articles, and prepositions will be the treatment targets.
The child was *not very cooperative* during assessment.	Often crying or whining, the child refused to name the pictures shown.
A variety of standardized and nonstandardized tests or procedures will be used in assessing the client's language.	Along with a conversational speech sample, the client's language will be evaluated with the Bankson Language Test, the Peabody Picture Vocabulary Test, and the Test for Examining Expressive Morphology.
The child with cleft palate and his or her family *need numerous services from an array of different specialists.*	The child with cleft palate and his or her family need services from many specialists including pediatricians, dentists, orthodontists, plastic surgeons, otologists, audiologists, speech-language pathologists, psychologists, and others.
Lack of treatment progress had *some negative effect* on the client's *emotionality*.	The client was disappointed because of lack treatment progress.

Note: In each of the correct examples, such general terms as "a variety of," "various," "numerous," "several," "many," "some," "positive effect," and so forth are replaced by specific terms.

A.2.11. USE DEFINITE, SPECIFIC, CONCRETE LANGUAGE

Incorrect	Write Correctly
The man with aphasia did not seem very happy during the treatment sessions.	
Voice therapy seems to have changed the life of Mr. Shreik.	
I will use any and all means of promoting response maintenance at home.	
The child did not want to be assessed.	
I will use many different procedures to assess the child's articulation.	
Stuttering has many kinds of effects on most aspects of life.	
A hearing impaired child with an active ear pathology needs a variety of professional services from many different specialists.	
The client was unfavorably disposed to continuing treatment next semester.	

A.2.12. ELIMINATE UNNECESSARY WORDS AND PHRASES

To be precise and more effective, eliminate unnecessary words and phrases.
They add nothing to the meaning.
Such unnecessary words and phrases as the following clutter sentences and lengthen them.

abilities (unless you distinguish it from action)
along the lines of
as a matter of fact
as far as ... is (are) concerned
at the present time
at this point in time
by means of
due to the fact that
experienced an inability
experienced great difficulty
for all intents and purposes
hands–on experience
in order to
in spite of the fact that
in the time frame
in the area of
in the event that
is considered to be
on account of the fact that
question as to whether
the fact of the matter is
the field of (communicative disorders, audiology, and so forth)
the type of (unless you describe different types)
unable to (in most cases)
until such time as
used for the purpose of
with regards to
with respect to
with reference to

A.2.12. ELIMINATE UNNECESSARY WORDS AND PHRASES

Find at least five unnecessary words and phrases that people use:

1.

2.

3.

4.

5.

Write both the wordy and the precise sentences.

Imprecise	Precise

Eliminate unnecessary words and phrases (continued)

Imprecise	Precise
In the time frame of an hour, a complete assessment may be made.	*In about an hour,* a complete assessment may be made.
Aphasia *is considered to be* a language disorder.	Aphasia is a language disorder.
We have much controversy *in the area of* language treatment.	We have much controversy in language treatment.
Reading, writing, and speaking *abilities* were affected.	Reading, writing, and speaking were affected.
The patient *experienced an inability* to produce speech.	The patient could not produce speech.
The tongue demonstrated weakness *with regards to* lateral strength.	The tongue demonstrated lateral weakness.
A mixed probe will be *the type of probe* administered.	A mixed probe will be administered.
If the client *is unable to* produce the word, the clinician will model it.	If the client cannot produce a word, the clinician will model it.
She *experienced great difficulty* speaking as demonstrated by slow, labored, and effortful speech.	Her speech was slow, labored, and effortful.
For all intents and purposes, assessment and diagnostics mean the same.	Assessment and diagnostics mean the same.
Treatment goals were not achieved *due to the fact that* the client missed several sessions.	Treatment goals were not achieved because the client missed several sessions.
On account of the fact that she was unemployed, she could not afford treatment.	Because she was unemployed, she could not afford treatment.
John won *in spite of the fact that* he was injured.	John won though he was injured.
We cannot offer any monetary rewards *at this point in time*.	We cannot offer any monetary rewards now.
At the present time, my case load is full.	Now my caseload is full.
I'm very busy *until such time as* the holidays are over.	I'm very busy until the holidays are over.
Our office is *used for the purposes of* distribution.	Our office is used for distribution.
In order to teach the morphologic features, I will model the correct responses.	To teach the morphologic features, I will model the correct responses.
The question as to whether children with articulation disorders have phonological disorders has been debated.	Whether children with articulation disorders have phonological disorders has been debated.
In the field of communicative disorders	In communicative disorders

Eliminate unnecessary words and phrases (continued)

Imprecise	Write Precisely
Modeling may be considered to be an effective stimulus control procedure.	
In the area of phonological disorders, we have many assessment procedures.	
Respiration, phonation, and articulation abilities were disturbed.	
The patient with laryngectomy experiences an inability to phonate normally.	
With regards to long–term effects, loud noise is detrimental to normal hearing.	
A single-subject design will be the type of design to be used in this study.	
When the client is unable to imitate a target response, I will use the shaping procedure.	
He experienced great difficulty in producing phonemes in sequence as demonstrated by his trial-and error movement of the articulators.	
Morphologic training was not initiated this semester due to the fact that the client did not meet the other targets.	
On account of the fact that they did not attend the IEP meetings, the parents could not be informed about the treatment targets.	
The client made excellent progress in spite of the fact that she had a severe articulation problem.	
The fact of the matter is that many untested theories confuse the clinician.	
Our waiting list is long at this point in time.	
At the present time, all the treatment targets have been achieved.	
Until such time as the interfering behaviors are controlled, language targets cannot be trained.	
Tokens may be used for the purposes of reinforcement.	
In order to assess the client's syntactic structures, a language sample was recorded.	
The client has the ability to speak fluently.	

Eliminate unnecessary words and phrases (continued)

He has *the ability to* lead the team.	He can lead the team.
It is good to get some *hands–on* experience in the workplace.	It is good to get some experience in the workplace.
During treatment, improvement *in terms of* the response rates was good.	During treatment, the response rates improved.
As far as the client's correct production of phonemes was concerned, the results were disappointing.	At home, the client did not (does not) correctly produce the phonemes.
In the event that Hector cannot complete the task, Sheila will take over.	If Hector cannot complete the task, Sheila will take over.
We will win *by means of* working harder.	We will win by working harder
He is a man who (*she is a woman who*) knows about religion.	He (She) knows about religion.
The clinician spoke *along the lines of* normal language development.	The clinician spoke about normal language development.
With reference to mild conductive hearing loss in infancy, it may cause language delay.	Mild conductive hearing loss in infancy may cause language delay.

Eliminate unnecessary words and phrases (continued)

Imprecise	Write Precisely
The researchers have investigated the question as to whether mild conductive hearing impairment in young children causes language delay.	
You can get some hands on experience in word processing at our computer lab.	
In terms of making a complete assessment, language samples are excellent.	
As far as the client's motivation for treatment is concerned, you should make a good judgment.	
In the time frame of 20 minutes, you should administer a probe.	
In the event that the treatment sessions cannot be held twice a week, a once-a-week schedule might be tried.	
Articulation was assessed by means of the Goldman-Fristoe Test of Articulation.	
She is a clinician who can treat patients with aphasia.	
The clinician worked along the lines of response maintenance.	
I think I have the ability to lead the team.	
The field of audiological practice is challenging and stimulating.	

A.2.13. AVOID REDUNDANT PHRASES

Redundant	Essential
future prospects	prospects
advance planning	planning
absolutely incomplete	incomplete
exactly identical	identical
repeat again	again
each and every	each *or* every
totally unique	unique
uniquely one of a kind	one of a kind *or* unique
reality as it is	reality
actual facts solid facts true facts	facts
famous and well-known	famous *or* well-known
goals and objectives	goals *or* objectives
three different kinds	three kinds
seven different varieties	seven varieties
four different types	four types
as of yet	yet
prison facilities church facilities hospital facilities	prison, church, hospital
crisis situation	crisis
problem situation	problem
prepay first	prepay *or* pay first
free gift	gift *or* free
positive growth	growth
bad weather conditions	bad weather
deteriorating economic conditions	deteriorating economy
deteriorating client response conditions	client's deteriorating responses
positive affirmative action	affirmative action
actively involved, actively looking	involved, looking
preconditions	conditions
unexpected surprise	surprise
successfully completed	completed
successfully avoided	avoided
make an effort to try	make an effort *or* try
advice and counsel	advice *or* counsel
necessary and essential	necessary *or* essential
fair and equitable	fair *or* equitable

A.2.13. AVOID REDUNDANT PHRASES

Find 10 redundant phrases used in everyday language.

Suggest the essential terms.

Redundant Phrases	Essential

A.2.14. AVOID WORDINESS

Wordy	Precise	Note
It seems to me that it is certainly very important to consider many factors in selecting treatment procedures for my clients.	I should consider many factors in selecting treatment procedures for my clients..	It is assumed that you will soon specify at least a few factors.
It became evident from my conversation with the parents of the child that they had a very difficult time to do what they were told to do because of their busy life style.	The parents of the child told me that they did not have time to conduct home treatment sessions.	
Although the client was certainly not negatively disposed to continuing the treatment for a reasonable amount of time, she finally decided to discontinue it.	The client discontinued the treatment, though she said she wanted to continue it.	The overused word *certainly* often suggests no certainty.
There were several crucial factors that led me to select these assessment procedures.	These assessment procedures were selected because of their known reliability, validity, and simplicity.	Often, the word *crucial* is an overstatement.
A variety of procedures will be used.	Many procedures will be used.	It is assumed that you specify the procedures in subsequent sentences.
A number of clients were treated.	Several clients were treated.	It is assumed that the exact number is unimportant.
Certain limitations of standardized tests make it imperative to carefully reconsider the whole issue of reliability and validity of assessment procedures.	Because of the limitations of standardized tests, we should reconsider the reliability and validity of assessment procedures.	It is assumed that you have specified the limitations.
It is not in the least inappropriate to offer the suggestion that cochlear implant may be a reasonably attractive method of aural rehabilitation that should not be rejected out of hand.	The option of cochlear implant should be considered.	The more precise statement says it positively as well.

A.2.14. AVOID WORDINESS

Wordy	Rewrite Precisely
In my judgment, it is reasonable to conclude that there are different types of aphasia though many symptoms are common to the different types.	
I personally think that it is not totally inappropriate to suggest that children with multiple misarticulations have a phonological disorder.	
I used two tests which were known to have a reasonable degree of reliability.	
It certainly seems to me that we need more treatment efficacy research.	
A variety of investigators have found it appropriate to suggest that both genetic and environmental factors play a causative role in stuttering.	
It is not unreasonable to suggest that we carefully consider all minimally attractive alternatives available to us as at this important juncture.	
It is certainly apparent to most competent clinicians that it is reasonably worthwhile to offer voice therapy to certain clients who may wish to consider it as an attractive alternative to surgical procedures.	
If one were to infer from these assessment data that the client has Broca's aphasia, the inference would certainly not seem totally inappropriate.	

A.2.15. KEEP RELATED WORDS TOGETHER

Intervening words that split related words can confuse the meaning.
Think which words of a sentence should be adjacent to each other.

Incorrect	Correct	Note
He ate seven hot dogs for lunch last Friday, and three more for dinner.	Last Friday, he ate seven hot dogs for lunch and three more for dinner.	
An unruly behavior of a child, if you do not control it, will prevent rapid progress in treatment.	Unless controlled, a child's unruly behavior will prevent rapid progress in treatment.	What prevents rapid progress?
Treatment of cluttering, because of limited research, is not well established.	Because of limited research, treatment of cluttering is not well established.	What is not well established?
Most clinicians, though they are keenly interested in it, are not well trained in the assessment of dysphagia.	Though they are keenly interested in it, most clinicians are not well trained in the assessment of dysphagia.	In what are the clinicians not well trained?

Note: Misplaced modifiers (see A.1.10) also create the same kind of problems as splitting related words.

A.2.15. KEEP RELATED WORDS TOGETHER

Incorrect	Write Correctly
Maintenance of target behaviors, if not carefully programmed, will not be achieved.	
In assessing phonological disorders, though many procedures may be appropriate, conversational speech is the most productive.	
Meeting the IEP goals within three months, even if I work hard and the child is regular for sessions, will be difficult.	
The selected target behaviors may be taught, assuming that the client will be regular for treatment sessions, in about 10 sessions.	
The final target of treatment, it has been suggested, is maintenance.	
The treatment procedure will include generalized reinforcers, to make it more effective.	

A.2.16. MAINTAIN PARALLELISM

Express parallel ideas in the same grammatical form. Parallel forms are forceful and concise. Parallelism is broken when two or more ideas are expressed in one form and the remaining idea is expressed in a different form.

Incorrect	Correct	Note
Children with language disorders tend to be deficient in their use of grammatic morphemes, syntactic structures, and *they also may have a limited vocabulary*.	Children with language disorders tend to be deficient in their use of grammatic morphemes, syntactic structures, and complex words.	The incorrect versions have a *nonparallel final clause*.
The hearing impaired child has difficulty speaking, reading, and *self-confidence*.	The hearing impaired child has difficulty speaking, reading, and in maintaining self-confidence.	
Disadvantages of primary reinforcers include satiation, dietary restriction, and *they also are difficult to administer to groups*.	Disadvantages of primary reinforcers include satiation, dietary restriction, and problematic group administration.	The correct versions restore parallelism to the final clause.
Parental reinforcement of target behaviors helps maintenance by *not* allowing extinction, strengthening the behaviors, and increasing their use in natural environments.	Parental reinforcement of target behaviors helps maintenance by *not* allowing extinction, by strengthening the behaviors, and by increasing their use in natural environments.	The incorrect version is nonparallel because the word *not* applies only to the first in the series. In the correct version, the repetition of *by* restores parallelism.

A.2.16. MAINTAIN PARALLELISM

Incorrect	Write Correctly
Many stutterers have suffered in the past because the therapists lacked adequate training, supervised experience, and the therapists' scientific knowledge of stuttering has been limited.	
Communicatively handicapped persons have difficulty talking, reading, and self-confidence.	
Some of the side effects of punishment are aggression, emotionality, and the client may also learn to punish others.	
Regulated breathing, developed by Azrin and associates (1975), which was researched by many other investigators, is known to be effective.	

A.2.17. AVOID DANGLING PHRASES

A phrase placed in a wrong position is called a dangling phrase.
For instance, a wrongly placed modifier may appear to modify the wrong word.
Dangling modifiers confuse meaning.
Also, a phrase that is better placed at the beginning of a sentence
may be left dangling at the end.

Incorrect	Correct	Note
The clinician selected children for treatment, *taking into consideration the eligibility criteria.*	*Taking into consideration the eligibility criteria,* the clinician selected children for treatment.	
Many undesirable effects of amplification have been eliminated, *using digital hearing aids.* (A dangling modifier)	1. *Using digital hearing aids,* many undesirable effects of amplification have been eliminated. 2. Researchers have shown that *digital hearing aids* eliminate many undesirable effects of amplification.	In most cases, fix the dangling phrases by moving them to an earlier position in the sentence
All children with communicative disorders will be offered treatment, *assuming that we have enough staff available to serve them.*	*Assuming that we have enough staff to serve them,* all children with communicative disorders will be offered treatment.	

A.2.17. AVOID DANGLING PHRASES

Incorrect	Write Correctly
I selected assessment procedures, giving much thought to reliability and validity.	
The problems of response maintenance may be handled, using parent training programs.	
Hearing will be tested, with an appropriately calibrated audiometer.	
Ten children will be selected for the study, all with a cochlear implant.	

A.2.18. AVOID SHIFTS WITHIN AND BETWEEN SENTENCES

Do not shift tense, voice, mood, and number within or between sentences.

Incorrect	Correct	Note
The clinician *was* well trained. She *knows* how to treat a variety of communicative disorders. Nevertheless, she *had* difficulty treating this particular client.	The clinician *was* well trained. She *knew* how to treat a variety of communicative disorders. Nevertheless, she *had* difficulty treating this particular client.	The incorrect version contain a shift in the tense. The correct version maintains the same past tense.
Van Riper first *developed* an eclectic theory and later a more integrative theory was also *proposed*.	Van Riper first *developed* an eclectic theory and later *proposed* a more integrative theory.	The incorrect version shows a shift from active to passive voice. The correct version maintains the active voice.
When *one* is reviewing the literature, *you* find that not many studies have been done on the issue.	When *one* is reviewing the literature, *one* finds that not many studies have been done on the issue.	The incorrect version shows a shift from first to third person. The correct version maintains the same pronoun form.
If a *client* does not attend at least 90 percent of the treatment sessions, *they* will not show significant improvement.	If a *client* does not attend at least 90 percent of the treatment sessions, *he* or *she* will not show significant improvement.	The incorrect version shifts from singular to plural. The correct version maintains the same number (singular).

A.2.18. AVOID SHIFTS WITHIN AND BETWEEN SENTENCES

Incorrect	Write Correctly
The client was highly motivated for treatment. Therefore, the progress *is* good.	
I will first train grammatic morphemes. Later, syntactic features also will be trained.	
When one considers treatment options, you find many options.	
A clinician who does not program maintenance will soon find that they have not completed the treatment.	
The review of the literature shows that this type of experiment has not been conducted. The review also has shown that it is difficult to control all the variables.	
The data suggested that the method was effective. The response rates indicates that maintenance also is enhanced.	

A.2.19. MAKE QUOTATIONS COUNT

Quotations are borrowed phrases.
Good quotations say something effectively and economically.
Therefore, do not quote descriptive and ordinary statements.

Descriptive and Ordinary	Rewritten Without Quotations	Note
Not all communicative disorders are related to environmental variables. Research has shown that "many genetic syndromes are associated with communicative disorders" (Brightly, 1993, p. 25).	Not all communicative disorders are related to environmental variables. Research has shown that several genetic syndromes also may be related to communicative disorders.	These quotations do not say anything worth quoting.
According to Qotme, "aphasia is a common communicative disorder found in the elderly" (1991, p. 9).	Among older people, aphasia is a common communicative disorder.	The writing is clearer without them.
Communicative disorders have a significant effect on the "social, occupational, and personal life of an individual" (Wisdon, 1993, p. 28).	Communicative disorders negatively affect an individual's personal, occupational, and social life (Wisdon, 1993).	Give reference to the source of information.
According to Surveyor, "roughly 10% of the population may have a communicative disorder" (1993, p. 18).	It is believed that 10% of the population may have a disorder of communication (Surveyor, 1993).	

A.2.19. MAKE QUOTATIONS COUNT

Descriptive and Ordinary	Rewrite Without Quotations
According to Verbose, "many school children have language disorders that go undetected" (1992, p. 50).	
Many researchers "have studied the relation between mild conductive hearing loss and language development" (Otis, 1993, p. 19).	
During hearing testing, "the clinician should mask the better ear" (Noisley, 1991, p. 567).	
According to Effecton, "some treatment procedures are effective while others are not" (1990, p. 20).	
Brimm has stated that "language acquisition is a complex process" (1989, p. 23).	

A.2.20. DO NOT OVERUSE QUOTATIONS

Do not use quotations to reduce the amount of your writing.
Unless a quote is memorable, paraphrase it and give credit.

Overuse	Judicious Use	Note
The study of language has shown "many rapid changes over the years" (Thomas, 1992, p. 90). In the 1940s "descriptive linguistics dominated the study of language" (TeNiel, 1985, p. 13). According to Thomas (1991), the focus shifted to "transformational generative grammar in the late 1950s and early 1960s" (p. 118). Then again in the 1970s, the focus was shifted to "the essence of language: meaning" (Wisdon, 1991, p. 50). Soon, however, this approach was abandoned in favor of a "new pragmatic approach" (Bomber, 1989, p. 120).	During the past few decades, the study of language has changed many times. In the 1940s, descriptive linguistics was the main approach to the study of language. Dissatisfied with a purely descriptive study, Chomsky (1957) and others in the late 1950s proposed a new transformational generative grammar approach. In the 1970s, those who disagreed with the purely theoretical grammar approach, proposed a new semantic view which focused on "the essence of language: meaning" (Wisdon, 1991, p. 50). Soon, this, too, was replaced by the newer pragmatic approach (Bomber, 1989).	Overuse of quotations tends to include unremarkable statements as well. Writing littered with ineffective quotes is difficult to read.

A.2.20. DO NOT OVERUSE QUOTATIONS

(In rewriting the passages, do not just eliminate the quotation marks. You should rephrase the quotations.)

Overuse	Rewrite With Fewer Quotations
Several forms of voice disorders are due to inappropriate behavior. According to Scream, "how you use your voice will determine whether you will have a healthy voice or not" (1992, p. 90). Loud (1987) also stated that "certain occupations pose high risk for voice disorders" (p. 13). Shout said a prudent person avoids "noisy places" (1988, p. 118).	
Either the right or the left ear may be tested first because "the selection is purely arbitrary" (Horton, 1992, p. 32). Research has not shown that it is "better to test one or the other ear first" (McClauey, 1993, p. 67). Most audiologists "begin testing at 1000 Hz, though the order in which the frequencies are tested may not be important" (Soundson, 1991, p. 45). Some audiologists "do not test at 125 Hz at all, while others do" (Southern, 1993, p. 22).	

A.2.21. DO NOT INCLUDE ISLANDS OF QUOTATIONS

Quotations should not stand alone in your writing.
Quotations should blend smoothly into your writing.

Incorrect	Correct	Note
Autism is a serious childhood disorder. It starts in early childhood. "Autistic children do not live in the world of their families, but in their own world of distorted fantasy" (Scitzmoore, 1993, p. 10). The disorder affects thought and language. "Autistic children are unable to form emotional bonds with their loved ones" (Sentiment, 1992, p. 15).	Autism is a serious childhood disorder. It starts in early childhood. Autistic children are not in touch with their surroundings as they seem to live "in their own world of distorted fantasy " (Scitzmoore, 1993, p. 10). The disorder affects thought, language, and emotional experience. According to Sentiment (1992), the autistic children are "unable to form emotional bonds with their loved ones" (p. 15).	You quote fewer words when you integrate quotations with your writing. In the correct version, no quotation stands alone. Such phrases as *according to ... as stated by* ... and (the author's name) *has written that* ... help blend a quotation with the main writing.

A.2.22. DO NOT BEGIN A SENTENCE WITH A QUOTATION

Begin sentences with your words.
Include quotations within or at the end of your sentence.

Incorrect	Correct
"Cleft palate speech is most readily recognized" (Milton, 1993, p. 20) because of its unique characteristics.	1. Because of its unique characteristics, "cleft palate speech is most readily recognized" (Milton, 1993, p. 20). 2. According to Milton (1993), "cleft palate speech is most readily recognized" (p. 20) because of its unique characteristics.
"In recent years, computerized audiometers have been developed to automatically control all aspects of pure tone air- and bone-conduction testing" (Robotson, 1993, p. 98); however, this does not mean that we "do not need audiologists who have a good clinical sense" (Robotson, 1993, p. 99).	In recent years, the administration of hearing tests has been computerized. However, as pointed out by Robotson (1993), we still need audiologists "who have a good clinical sense" (p. 99).

A.2.21. DO NOT INCLUDE ISLANDS OF QUOTATIONS

Incorrect	Write Correctly
Multiple misarticulations suggest a need for a phonological process analysis. "A process analysis helps the clinician see order in what might appear to be a collection of random errors" (Godsen, 1992, p. 45). Several methods of phonological analysis are available. "The clinician should select the one that is simple to use and comprehensive in its analysis" (Nixon, 1990, p. 10).	

A.2.22. DO NOT BEGIN A SENTENCE WITH A QUOTATION

Incorrect	Write Correctly
"Audiometers alone, no matter how advanced, will not diagnose hearing impairment" (Torkin, 1993, p. 32). It is the clinician's expert interpretation of results that leads to a clinical diagnosis. "No mechanical device is a substitute for good clinical sense" (Barkin, 1990, p. 551).	
"Specific language disorder often is not associated with an identifiable cause" (Barney, 1992, p. 40). The child may be normal in every respect except for delayed language. "It is hypothesized that specific language delay may have a genetic basis" (Tomokin, 1993, p. 22).	

A.2.23. USE QUOTATION AND PUNCTUATION MARKS CORRECTLY

Enclose all direct quotations within two double quotations marks ("and").
Use single quotation marks ('and') to enclose a quotation within a quotation.
In most cases, place the punctuation mark **within** the quotation mark.
Double check for missing quotation marks at the beginning or the ending of quotations.

Incorrect	Correct	Note
The clinician said, "Good job".	The clinician said, "Good job."	The first two incorrect versions have the punctuation mark outside the quotation marks.
I will say "wrong", and then mark the incorrect response on the sheet.	I will say "wrong," and then mark the incorrect response on the sheet.	
He said that he was "sorry for what happened.	He said that he was "sorry for what happened."	The next two have missing quotation marks.
According to Soundson, hearing impairment costs billions of dollars to the nation's health care system" (1993, p. 9).	According to Soundson, "hearing impairment costs billions of dollars to the nation's health care system" (1993, p. 9).	In scientific writing, all quotations are referenced.

A.2.24. DO NOT OVERUSE QUOTATION MARKS

Do not enclose the following within quotation marks;
instead, underline them or italicize them:

   Book and journal titles
   Technical terms, terms of special emphasis, and sarcastic terms
   Slang

Incorrect	Correct	Note
1. "Aphasia: A clinical approach"	*Aphasia: A clinical approach*	A book title, italicized.
2. "Journal of Audiology"	<u>Journal of Audiology</u>	A journal name, underlined.
3. "Dysphonia" means disordered voice.	*Dysphonia* means disordered voice. **Dysphonia** means disordered voice.	A technical term, defined.
4. This gobbledygook is promoted as an "explanation" of phonological acquisition.	This gobbledygook is promoted as an *explanation* of phonological acquisition.	Sarcasm.
5. She is "into" the whole language.	She uses the *whole language* approach.	Slang. *Slang is omitted in formal writing.*

Exception: The titles of articles, papers, theses, and so forth are neither enclosed within quotation marks nor italicized or underlined.

A.2.23. USE QUOTATION AND PUNCTUATION MARKS CORRECTLY

Incorrect	Write Correctly
Mrs. Aktsungfoong added that her husband is "stubborn" and "difficult to manage".	
The parents said that their son is "delighted", "very pleased", and "impressed" with the services.	
One expert stated that remediating pragmatic language disorders is the most important treatment target".	

A.2.24. DO NOT OVERUSE QUOTATION MARKS

Incorrect	Write Correctly
"Introduction to Audiology" by Matson	
"Journal of Speech and Hearing Research."	
"Congenital disorder" is a disorder noticed at the time of birth or soon thereafter.	
Does he think that rail walking is "therapy" for children with motor speech disorders?	
Some clinicians are "flying by the seat of their pants."	

A.2.25. GIVE REFERENCES FOR ALL DIRECT QUOTATIONS

In scientific writing, all direct quotations should include the following:

- the last name of the author or authors
- the year of publication
- the number of the page or pages on which the quotation is found

Incorrect	Correct	Note
According to Confusius, stuttering is due to "a terrible confusion between who you are and what you want to be."	According to Confusius (1993), stuttering is due to "a terrible confusion between who you are and what you want to be" (p. 37).	The incorrect version includes neither the year of publication nor the page number.
Mixtupton recommended that "children with phonological disorders should be separated from those with a mere articulation disorder" (1993).	Mixtupton recommended that "children with phonological disorders should be separated from those with a mere articulation disorder" (1993, p. 23).	The incorrect version includes the year of publication, but omits the page number.
It has been stated that "chronic and excessively loud speech is detrimental to healthy voice."	It has been stated that "chronic and excessively loud speech is detrimental to healthy voice" (Louden, 1992, p. 10).	The worst of the three, this incorrect version omits the author's name, year of publication, and the page number.
Though stuttering persons may show some excessive anxiety, it is "often associated with speech, and, therefore, there is no evidence for a "trait anxiety" in most stutterers" (Angst, 1991, p. 67).	Though stuttering persons may show some excessive anxiety, it is "often associated with speech, and, therefore, there is no evidence for a 'trait anxiety' in most stutterers" (Angst, 1991, p. 67).	A phrase with double quotation marks within a quotation is enclosed within single quotation marks.
Although found in all societies, "the incidence of cleft palate varies across different racial groups, suggesting the importance of genetic factors in its etiology" (Geneson, 1990, p. 10-11).	Although found in all societies, "the incidence of cleft palate varies across different racial groups, suggesting the importance of genetic factors in its etiology" (Geneson, 1990, pp. 10-11).	The correct version shows the page on which the quotation begins and the page on which it ends. p. for one page. pp. for two or more pages. Both in lower case.

There are different methods of placing the name, the year, and the page number.

The period is placed only after the parenthetical closure, not before or after the quotation marks.

A.2.25. GIVE REFERENCES FOR ALL DIRECT QUOTATIONS

Invent the information that is necessary to write correctly.

Incorrect	Write Correctly
According to Loveson, language delay is due to "many factors but none can be directly traced to lack of parental love for the child."	
Boontenthorpe has written that "adults who have strokes and aphasia show remarkable spontaneous recovery within three to six months of onset" (1993).	
It has been stated that "a single, loud scream can damage the vocal cords."	
A neglected cause of hearing impairment is "the types of food we eat; it is possible that "pesticide–laced grains and fruits" are a source of cochlear damage in some cases" (Peston, 1991, p. 67).	
Recent developments in cochlear implants have "made it possible for many deaf children to begin their aural rehabilitation early in life" (Coplant, 1990, p. 15-16).	

A.2.26. REPRODUCE QUOTATIONS EXACTLY

Make quotations identical to the original in words, spelling, and punctuation.
Reproduce errors as they are in the original with the insertion of the word [*sic*], italicized (or underlined), and placed within brackets.

A Quotation With an Error in It	Note
Numbasa's description of language as a mental phenomenon "that can be studied only by some powerfil [*sic*] intuitive procedures" was especially appealing to clinicians who had based their treatment procedures on intuition.	In the quotation, the italicized word [sic] suggests that in the original, the word *powerful* is misspelled.

A.2.27. INTEGRATE QUOTATIONS OF LESS THAN 40 WORDS WITH THE TEXT

Incorrect (Unintegrated)	Correct	Note
Numbasa defined language as: "A cognitive ability to synthesize and symbolize mental experience and to represent this experience in patterns of sounds, words, and sentences following linguistic rules that are innately given" (1971, p. 95)	Numbasa defined language as "a cognitive ability to synthesize and symbolize mental experience and to represent this experience in patterns of sounds, words, and sentences following linguistic rules that are innately given" (1971, p. 95).	Only quotations of 40 words or more are set off from the rest of the text. See A.2.28.

A.2.28. *BLOCK* QUOTATIONS WHEN THEY HAVE 40 WORDS OR MORE

- A quotation set apart from the text is a block quotation.
- Type quotations of 40 words or more as block quotations.
- Add an extra line (resulting in triple space) before and after a block quotation.
- Type the entire quotation indented five spaces from the left margin.
- Indent the first line of the second (and subsequent) paragraphs five more spaces.
- Do not use quotation marks.
- However, place within *double quotation marks* a quotation within a block quotation.
- After the quotation, type the page number of the quotation within parentheses.
- Do not type a period after the closing parenthesis.

A.2.26. REPRODUCE QUOTATIONS EXACTLY

Quotation With an Error in It	Quote It Appropriately
Dinson (1987) said that "language is not to be confused with what people say, because language is a metal tool of imagination" (p. 40).	

A.2.27. INTEGRATE QUOTATIONS OF LESS THAN 40 WORDS WITH THE TEXT

Incorrectly Arranged Quotation	Integrate the Quote With Text
Galle (1993) stated that: Every child who learns to speak his or her language is a scientist who tests alternative hypotheses about the nature of language. The spoken language the child hears is the data for hypothesis testing. (p. 23) This statement made a profound impact on the study of language and its natural acquisition. This statement also is popular with many clinicians.	

Block quotations (continued)

Block Quotation	Note
In his powerful explanation of language intervention, Mumbasa (1991) has stated the following: Language intervention is a process of unleashing powerful but painfully hidden though unconsciously active communicative potential. It is not a process of teaching "communicative behaviors"—an empty phrase that is popular these days. The goals of language intervention include transcendental self-actualization, cognitive reorganization, and remodeling of perceptual-emotive reality. These goals are most successfully met by forging a unity between the unknown demands made on the individual and his or her hidden but striving communicative potential. If the process of language intervention as described in this book sounds mysterious, it is because the process is mysterious. A successful clinician has an innate ability to solve this mystery. (p. 19)	The first line of the block quotation is indented five spaces from the left margin. There are no quotation marks. A quote within a block quotation is enclosed within double quotation marks. The entire quotation is double-spaced. The second paragraph is indented five more spaces. Two spaces are given before the first parenthesis is started to enclose the page number. There is no period after the closing parenthesis.

A.2.28. *BLOCK* QUOTATIONS WHEN THEY HAVE 40 WORDS OR MORE

Quotation of More Than 40 Words	Arrange It Properly
Confidon (1992) has stated that "the root cause of stuttering is lack of self-confidence. Fluent speech is a function of strong self-confidence because we are not fluent when we are not sure of ourselves. When we know what we want to say and how to say it, we are generally fluent. Therefore, to make stuttering persons speak fluently, we must find ways of enhancing their self-confidence" (pp. 35-36). All clinicians should consider this powerful explanation of stuttering in planning treatment for stuttering persons.	

A.2.29. SHOW CORRECTLY THE CHANGES IN QUOTATIONS

When you omit words from a sentence within a quotation, insert three ellipsis marks (...).

When you omit words between sentences, insert four ellipsis marks (....).

Do not insert ellipsis marks at the beginning and end of a quotation even when it begins or ends in midsentence.

If you insert words into a quotation, enclose them within brackets.

Underline or italicize the words *you* emphasize that were not emphasized in the original.

Next to the underlined or italicized words, type the words [italics added] within brackets.

Changed Quotation	Note
Bluff has stated that "stuttering cannot be measured by... merely counting dysfluencies. Stuttering and dysfluencies are not to be confused.... It [stuttering] is more than *mere dysfluencies*" [italics added] (1993, p. 58).	Omitted words within a sentence indicated: *by... merely* Omitted words between sentences indicated: *confused.... It* (a period, three dots, and two spaces) Inserted word bracketed: *It* [stuttering] *is*

A.2.29. SHOW CORRECTLY THE CHANGES IN QUOTATIONS

Changed Quotation	Rewrite Correctly
Snuff has stated that "Voice disorders are not only a product of various medical pathologies (words omitted) but also a product of certain life styles. Therefore, clinicians should take a careful and detailed history of the client (words omitted at the end of the sentence). Information obtained through history is invaluable in planning treatment *for voice clients* (added words). They (*the clinicians*: added words) *should not hesitate to probe the client's life style"* (italics not in the original) (1990, p. 50).	

A.2.30. USE LATIN ABBREVIATIONS ONLY IN PARENTHETICAL CONSTRUCTIONS

In nonparenthetical sentences, use their English equivalents:

Abbreviation	English Equivalent
etc.	and so forth
e. g.,	for example
i.e.,	that is
viz.,	namely
vs.	versus, against
	Exception: Use the abbreviation v for versus when referring to court cases: *The historic Brown v Board of Education ruling has been upheld.*

Exception:

Use the Latin abbreviation et al., *which means "and others" in parenthetical and nonparenthetical writing.*

Do not use Latin abbreviations in conversational speech.

Incorrect	Correct
Pictures, objects, line drawings, etc., will be used as stimuli.	Pictures, objects, line drawings, and so forth, will be used as stimuli.
Various reinforcers, e.g., tokens, stickers, and points, will be used as reinforcers.	Various reinforcers, for example, tokens, stickers, and points, will be used as reinforcers.
The basic continuous reinforcement schedule, i.e., the FR1, may be used.	The basic continuous reinforcement schedule, that is, the FR1, may be used.
Certain variables, *viz.,* motivation, severity of the disorder, and intelligence are known to influence the treatment outcome.	Certain variables, namely, motivation, severity of the disorder, and intelligence are known to influence the treatment outcome.
Nativism vs. empiricism is a historical topic of discussion.	Nativism versus empiricism is a historical topic of discussion.

A.2.30. USE LATIN ABBREVIATIONS ONLY IN PARENTHETICAL CONSTRUCTIONS

Take note of an exception, however.

Incorrect	Write Correctly
Interjections, prolongations, repetitions, etc. are among the types of dysfluencies.	
Certain types of newer hearing aids, e.g., the digital aids, can reduce background noise.	
Neural hearing loss, i.e., the type of loss with nerve damage, is difficult to treat surgically.	
Many variables, viz., heredity, environmental toxicity, and maternal alcoholism can cause mental retardation.	
Behaviorism vs. cognitivism is a good topic for debate.	
The Brown versus the Board of education ruling forced racial integration in public schools.	

A.2.31. AVOID EUPHEMISM

Euphemistic expressions disguise negative meanings.
Such expressions falsely suggest neutral or positive meanings.
Euphemistic writing can be dishonest.

Euphemistic	Direct
Because of poor progress, the family will be *counseled out* of our services.	1. Because of poor progress, the family will be dismissed from our services. 2. Because of poor progress, we recommended to the family that our services be discontinued.
The client is *communicatively challenged*.	1. The client has a communicative disorder. 2. The client has an articulation problem.
The child comes from an *economically deprived* background.	The child comes from a poor family.
The child is *mentally other-abled*.	The child is mentally retarded.

A.2.32. AVOID JARGON

Jargon is a technical or specialized term; sometimes it is unavoidable.
Do not overuse jargon.
When necessary, describe what jargon means in everyday language.
When you write to persons without technical knowledge, describe everything in nontechnical terms.
When writing to technical audiences, retain the technical terms.

Jargon	Plain
The child's *linguistic competence* is limited.	The child's *language* is limited.
Use an *FR2 schedule* to reinforce correct responses at home.	Reinforce *every other correct response* at home.
In using your hearing aid, you should learn to control the *intensity of the signal*.	In using your hearing aid, you should learn to control the *volume*.
The child's *MLU* is limited.	The child speaks in *short phrases or sentences*.
The woman has *anomia*.	The woman has naming difficulties.

A.2.31. AVOID EUPHEMISM

Euphemistic	Write More Directly
The student was counseled out of the major.	
The child comes from an underprivileged family.	
The man is physically challenged.	
Today, the garbologist did not collect the trash.	
I bought a previously owned car.	

A.2.32. AVOID JARGON

Jargon	Write in Plain Language
The boy has a severe problem in correctly positioning his articulators.	
The patient has agrammatism.	
The woman has aphonia.	

A.2.33. AVOID CLICHÉS

Clichés are overused and dull expressions.
Replace clichés with more appropriate words.

Cliché	Simple and Direct	Note
We do not have too many *tried-and-true* treatment techniques.	We do not have too many *proven* treatment techniques.	The word *proven* is more acceptable for this kind of writing.
Though he recently had a stroke, the patient was *fit as a fiddle*.	Though he recently had a stroke, the patient was in good health.	An everyday term is more appropriate than the cliché.
Treating patients with laryngectomy is not her *cup of tea*.	1. She does not enjoy treating patients with laryngectomy. 2. She does not know how to treat patients with laryngectomy.	Some clichés mask multiple meanings.

A.2.34. AVOID COLLOQUIAL OR INFORMAL EXPRESSIONS

The rule applies to scientific and professional writing.

Informal	Formal	Note
If the client *can't* imitate, I will use the shaping method..	If the client *cannot* imitate, I will use the shaping method.	Avoid informal contractions.
Continuous reinforcement *won't* be used.	Continuous reinforcement *will not* be used.	
The researcher *felt* that the procedure was effective.	The researcher *thought* that the procedure was effective.	Avoid such subjective terms as *felt* unless the reference is to feelings.
The clinician should *get across* the idea that maintenance treatment is important.	The clinician should *point out* that maintenance treatment is important.	Colloquial
The clinician *came up* with a dysphagia assessment procedure.	The clinician *developed* a dysphagia assessment procedure.	

A.2.33. AVOID CLICHÉS

Cliché	Write in Simple and Direct Words
The child is bored to tears with therapy.	
The initial progress gave the client a shot in the arm.	
The stuttering child is sick and tired of teasing from her friends.	

A.2.34. AVOID COLLOQUIAL OR INFORMAL EXPRESSIONS

Informal	Formal
The client just wouldn't imitate the modeled stimulus.	
The clinician hadn't prepared the stimulus materials.	
I feel that the client's hoarseness of voice is due to vocal nodules.	
In counseling the parents of a child with a hearing loss, you should get across the idea that the early intervention is important.	
The clinician cooked up a novel method of evoking the /r/.	

A.3. COMMONLY MISUSED WORDS AND PHRASES

Use the following words or phrases correctly. Know the differential meaning of the words that are often confused.

A.3.1. AFFECT AND EFFECT

Use *affect* as a verb, *effect* as a noun

Incorrect	Correct
Many researchers have studied the masking noise *affect* on stuttering.	Many researchers have studied the masking noise *effect* on stuttering.
The treatment *affect* was studied.	The treatment *effect* was studied.
The treatment *effected* the behavior.	The treatment *affected* the behavior.
How did the variable *effect* the outcome?	How did the variable *affect* the outcome?

A.3.2. ALTERNATE AND ALTERNATIVE

Alternate means occurring or succeeding by turns; to alternate is to shift from one to the other. *Alternative* suggests a choice between two possibilities.

Incorrect	Correct	Note
I will use the alternative treatments design.	I will use the alternating treatments design.	You shift from one treatment to the other.
Alternative current	Alternating current	Current reverses its direction at regular intervals.
I will take the alternative route.	I will take the alternate route.	The person took the other route.
The only alternate to treatment is continued stuttering.	The only alternative to treatment is continued stuttering.	The statement says there is only one choice.

A.3.3. ALLUSION AND ILLUSION

Use *illusion* to refer to an unreal image and *allusion* to suggest an indirect reference.

Incorrect	Correct
She made an illusion to the new theory of voice production.	She made an allusion to the new theory of voice production.
The ghost he thought he saw was merely an allusion.	The ghost he thought he saw was merely an illusion.

A.3. COMMONLY MISUSED WORDS AND PHRASES

A.3.1. AFFECT AND EFFECT

Incorrect	Write Correctly
The *affect* of environmental deprivation on language acquisition is significant.	
This study on the *affect* of aphasia treatment was poorly designed.	
Modeling *effected* the target response.	
How does the parental dysfluency rate *effect* the child's stuttering?	

A.3.2. ALTERNATE AND ALTERNATIVE

Incorrect	Write Correctly
It leaves me with no alternate.	
You can alternative the two probe procedures.	

A.3.3. ALLUSION AND ILLUSION

Incorrect	Write Correctly
He made an illusion to an emerging trend in the treatment of dysarthria.	
The treatment effects reported in the study were merely an allusion.	

A.3.4. AND/OR

Do not write *and/or*. Rewrite the sentence.

Incorrect	Correct
Pictures and/or objects will be used to evoke the target behaviors.	Pictures, objects, or both will be used to evoke the target behaviors.
Speech-language pathologists and/or psychologists may assess patients with aphasia.	Speech-language pathologists, psychologists, or both may assess patients with aphasia.

A.3.5. FARTHER AND FURTHER

Use *farther* to refer to distance. Use *further* to refer to time or quantity.

Incorrect	Correct
She walked further than any person.	She walked farther than any person.
I sent the parents a farther notice of an IEP meeting.	I sent the parents a further notice of an IEP meeting.
Farthermore, the client was often late.	Furthermore, the client was often late.

A.3.6. INCIDENCE AND PREVALENCE

Incidence refers to the future occurrence of an event in a population.

    (How many normally speaking children will begin to stutter?)

Prevalence refers to the current existence; you take a head count.

    (How many children in the city have a hearing impairment?)

Incorrect	Correct	Note
The incidence of stuttering in the population of the United States is about 2 million.	The incidence of stuttering in the population of the United States is about 1 percent.	Incidence of stuttering refers to the number of people who are expected to stutter.
The prevalence of hearing impairment is about 10 percent.	There are about 2,000 children in the city who have a hearing impairment. Such a high prevalence of hearing impairment requires the services of additional educators of the deaf.	Prevalence refers to the total number of persons who already have a problem or a disorder.

A.3.4. AND/OR

Incorrect	Write Correctly
The father and/or the mother of the client will be trained in response maintenance.	
Language disorders and/or phonological disorders may coexist with stuttering.	

A.3.5. FARTHER AND FURTHER

Incorrect	Write Correctly
New York is further than you think.	
It is not sufficient to establish the target behaviors. The clinician should do farther work on maintenance.	

A.3.6. INCIDENCE AND PREVALENCE

Incorrect	Write Correctly
The incidence of aphasia in the state is more than 100,000.	
The prevalence of language disorders in the school-age children in the city is about 10 percent.	

A.3.7. INTER- AND INTRA-

Inter- means *between* or *among*.
Intra- means *within*.

Incorrect	Correct	Note
The intraobserver reliability index is based on the observation of two graduate students.	Intraobserver reliability is based on two observations of the experimenter.	The same person made two observations. Therefore, the observations give an index of *intra*observer reliability.
The interobserver reliability index is based on the experimenter's two observations.	The interobserver reliability index is based on the observation of two experts.	Two persons made observations of the same event. Therefore, the observations give an index of *inter*observer reliability.

A.3.8. LATTER AND LATER

Latter means the second or the last of a group of things; it is the one that comes after but without a specific reference to time.
Later has a specific reference to time: after a specified time.

Incorrect	Correct	Note
Latter I will work on maintenance.	Later I will work on maintenance.	Your work on maintenance comes later in time.
Treatment is first, probes are later.	Treatment is first, probes are latter.	Probing is a subsequent procedure. It is done whenever treatment is implemented.

A.3.7. INTER- AND INTRA-

Incorrect	Correct
I will establish the intraobserver reliability by correlating my observations with those of another observer.	
The experimenter established interobserver reliability index by correlating two of her observations.	

A.3.8. LATER AND LATTER

Incorrect	Correct
I will do it latter.	
The first procedure is to clear the wax in the ear. A latter procedure is to test the hearing.	

A.3.9. SECONDLY AND THIRDLY

Avoid this usage. Write: First, Second, Third, and so forth.

Not Preferred	Preferred	Note
First, I will assess the client. Secondly, I will select the target behaviors. Thirdly, I will prepare the stimulus materials.	First, I will assess the client. Second, I will select the target behaviors. Third, I will prepare the stimulus materials.	Some write *firstly*, but it is worse than *secondly* and *thirdly*.

A.3.10. SINCE AND BECAUSE

The word *since* often is misused.
Use *since* to suggest temporal (time) sequence, as in *Since the introduction of in-the-ear hearing aids, social acceptability of hearing aid usage has increased.*
Use *because* to suggest causation.

Incorrect	Correct	Note
Since the stimulus pictures are ambiguous, the responses are not certain.	Because the stimulus pictures are ambiguous, the responses are not certain.	Uncertain responses are due to ambiguous pictures.

A.3.11. USE UNUSUAL SINGULARS AND PLURALS CORRECTLY

Incorrect	Correct	Note
Data *is* presented in Table 1.	Data are Presented in Table 1.	*Data* is a plural word
The datum *are* interesting.	The datum is interesting.	*Datum* is singular
The *phenomena* of vocal abuse is widespread.	The phenomenon of vocal abuse is widespread.	*Phenomena* is a plural word.
These *phenomenon* have been recorded.	These phenomena have been recorded.	*Phenomenon* is singular.
The *loci* of stuttering is well known.	The loci of stuttering are well known.	*Loci* is a plural word.
The year of publication should be in *parenthesis*.	The year of publication should be in *parentheses*.	*Parentheses* is plural.
I wrote a theses.	I wrote a thesis.	*Theses* is plural.

A.3.9. SECONDLY AND THIRDLY

Not Preferred	Preferred
First, I will instruct the client on what he or she should do. Secondly, I will place the headphones on the client. Thirdly, I will begin hearing testing.	

A.3.10. SINCE AND BECAUSE

Incorrect	Write Correctly
Since the auditory discrimination procedure was not effective, I shifted to production training.	
Since the child is not cooperative, automatic audiologic assessment procedures are necessary.	

A.3.11. USE UNUSUAL SINGULARS AND PLURALS CORRECTLY

Incorrect	Write Correctly
Her data *is* quite complex.	
Scientists cannot control the various natural phenomenon.	
The phenomena of central auditory processing is a mystery.	
The loci of vocal nodules is variable within a small range.	

Note to Student Writers

Examples on the previous pages sample only a small number of commonly misused words and phrases. Use this page to write down additional examples of such words and phrases. Practice correct usage of those words and phrases.

PART B

SCIENTIFIC WRITING

B.1. PRINCIPLES OF SCIENTIFIC WRITING

Printed Notes	Class Notes

There are many forms of scientific writing.

The most common form is a research paper.

Scientific papers have somewhat rigid

formats.

Different scientific journals have their

specific formats.

Scientific writing is:

- related to data, research, or theory

- direct

- precise

- objective

- organized according to an accepted
  format.

B.2. WRITING WITHOUT BIAS

Printed Notes	Class Notes

An important skill to acquire is *writing without bias*.

Scientific writing should be free from racial, cultural, ethnic, social, economic, and gender-related biases.

Negative connotations about disabilities, unless such connotations are a matter of scientific study, also should be avoided.

Scientific writing avoids stereotypic language about sexes, individuals, and ethnic groups.

Scientific writing makes reference to ethnic, racial, and other cultural factors only when:

- those factors themselves are the subject of a study

- the knowledge of such factors are necessary to understand the results of a study or issues on hand

Printed Notes	**Class Notes**

Necessary reference to gender, culture, ethnicity, and race are made in:

- nonevaluative and non offensive language

- terms that groups use to refer to themselves

Gender bias is the most frequent problem.

Implied or direct negative reference to disabilities also is a frequent problem.

Important: Note that biases are not just a problem in scientific writing.

They are a problem in:

- all writing

- conversational speech

- media expressions

Printed Notes	Class Notes

Your speech and all forms of writing should
be free from biases.

The APA *Manual* has guidelines on writing
without racial, gender-related, and other
kinds of biases. Study those guidelines. On
the following pages, you will find examples
of and exercises for writing without bias.

B.2.1. WRITE WITHOUT GENDER BIAS

Terms That Suggest Bias	Appropriate Use	Note
man	Use only when you refer to a male person	
mankind	*humankind, humans, people*	
he his (other male referents)	*he or she* [but not *he/she*, nor *(s)he*] *his or her*	Of course, the male referents are fine if the reference is restricted to male persons.
Animals share only a part of man's capacity for communication.	Animals share only a part of humans' capacity for communication.	
The recent scientific achievements of mankind are unparalleled in history.	1. The recent scientific achievements of men and women are unparalleled in history. 2. The recent scientific achievements of humans are unparalleled in history.	
The child is not alone in his language acquisition process. He gets significant help from his caregivers.	1. The children are not alone in their language acquisition process. They get significant help from their caregivers. 2. The child is not alone in his or her language acquisition process. He or she gets significant help from caregivers.	The excessive use of *he or she* makes the writing cumbersome to read. Use plural pronouns as in the first example.
The child may be referred to a pediatrician with the expectation that he will follow up on the recommendations.	The child may be referred to a pediatrician with the expectation that she or he will follow up on the recommendations.	Alternate the order in which you write *he or she (she or he) woman or man (man or woman)*

B.2.1. WRITE WITHOUT GENDER BIAS

Incorrect	Write Correctly
The stuttering client is typically frustrated with *his* attempts at communication.	
Mankind has known about aphasia for a long time, though the treatment methods were unknown.	
Refer the client to a biotechnician. *He* will make a prosthetic device for the client.	
Hearing loss in old age affects a *man's* social behavior.	
The dialect of *black* persons has a unique and rich history.	Note: Substitute the word *black* for the phrase now preferred.

B.2.2. WRITE WITHOUT PREJUDICIAL REFERENCE TO DISABILITIES

Describe disabilities objectively.
Avoid sentimental or evaluative terms.
Put people first, not their disability.
Do not use disabilities to suggest metaphoric meanings.

Incorrect	Correct	Note
The man was a *victim* of laryngectomy.	The man had laryngectomy.	Avoid such terms as *victim* and *suffers from* because they suggest negative evaluations
The child *suffers from* severe articulation problems.	The child has a severe articulation disorder.	
The man with aphasia is *crippled*.	The man with aphasia has hemiplegia.	
The *stutterer* could not order in restaurants.	1. Mr. Jones, who stutters, could not order in restaurants. 2. A person who stutters has difficulty ordering in restaurants.	The correct versions put the persons first, not their disabilities.
The child *stutterer* did not ask questions in the classroom.	1. The child, because of her stuttering, did not ask questions in the classroom. 2. The child, who stutters, did not ask questions in the classroom.	
The *aphasic* did not recall the names.	1. The woman with aphasia did not recall the names. 2. The aphasic person did not recall the names.	The term *aphasic* is not a noun; it is an adjective.
The *wheelchaired* need access to our classrooms and clinics.	Persons in wheelchairs need access to our classrooms and clinics.	
Supervisors are *blind* to our day-to-day problems.	1. Supervisors do not see our day-to-day problems. 2. Supervisors do not appreciate our day-to-day problems.	Metaphoric use of a disability.

B.2.2. WRITE WITHOUT PREJUDICIAL REFERENCE TO DISABILITIES

Incorrect	Write Correctly
The child was a victim of bilateral clefts of the hard palate.	
The woman suffers from dementia.	
The disabled person is crippled.	
Blind and deaf children need special methods to learn communication.	
The teachers' plea for more computers fell on deaf ears.	
This aphasic has lost her speech.	
The deaf child learned to use the sign language.	
The stutterer agreed to come for treatment.	
The dysarthric had prosodic problems.	
The paraplegic need appropriate access to buildings.	
The traffic problem is crippling.	

Note to Student Writers

Local or national television news is not entirely free from biased reporting. If you watch a few news episodes critically, you will be surprised at the amount of biased reporting that exists.

Biased oral or written expressions suggesting negative connotations regarding people who are poor, less educated, and those living in rural areas also are common. Study selected broadcast programs and newspaper articles to find examples of such expressions.

B.3. FORMAT OF SCIENTIFIC WRITING

B.3.1. GIVE CORRECT MARGINS

Margins should be 1 1/2 inches (4 cm) on the top, bottom, right, and left of every page.
The wide margin space is used to edit papers or write comments. Therefore, make sure you use
the specified margins on all papers you submit.

	Top 1.5" margin	
Left 1.5" margin		Right 1.5" margin
	Bottom 1.5" margin	

B.3.2. LINE SPACING

Double Space	Triple Space	Single Space
title page entire paper all headings all text quotations tables figure legends reference lists	before starting a major heading. before and after a blocked quotation.	no portion of the paper *Exception:* **The final versions of clinical reports.** These are always single-spaced.

B.3.3. USE ACCEPTABLE COMPUTER PRINTERS AND TYPEFACES

Acceptable	Unacceptable	Note
Letter–quality printers Laser printers Ink jet printers	Dot matrix printers Exotic and ornamental typefaces Cursive typefaces Condensed type	Use typefaces that are clear and easy to read.

B.3.4. DO NOT OVERUSE BOLDFACE

Use bold to	Do not use bold to	Note
highlight technical or other important terms. highlight headings and subheadings.	highlight quotations.	Do not use bold when italics are needed (e.g., book and journal titles).

B.3.5. USE THE RECOMMENDED TYPE SIZE

The same size letters may look larger or smaller, depending on the typeface.
For instance, 12 point Times Roman may be smaller than 12 point Geneva.
Use your judgment.

Recommended Size	Unacceptable	Note
12 point	Very large or very small sizes	See how the printed page looks and make judgments.

B.3.6. USE ACCEPTABLE PAPER

Acceptable	Unacceptable	Note
For drafts: Ordinary computer or copy paper For the final submission: Letter size (8 1/2 X 11"), white, nonerasable, unlined bond paper with 25% cotton content (letterhead quality)	For the final submission: typical computer paper or copy paper (These are not 25% cotton bond.)	If cost is a factor, talk to your instructor and get a waiver.

B.3.7. TYPE CORRECTLY THE TITLE PAGE OF A PAPER FOR PUBLICATION

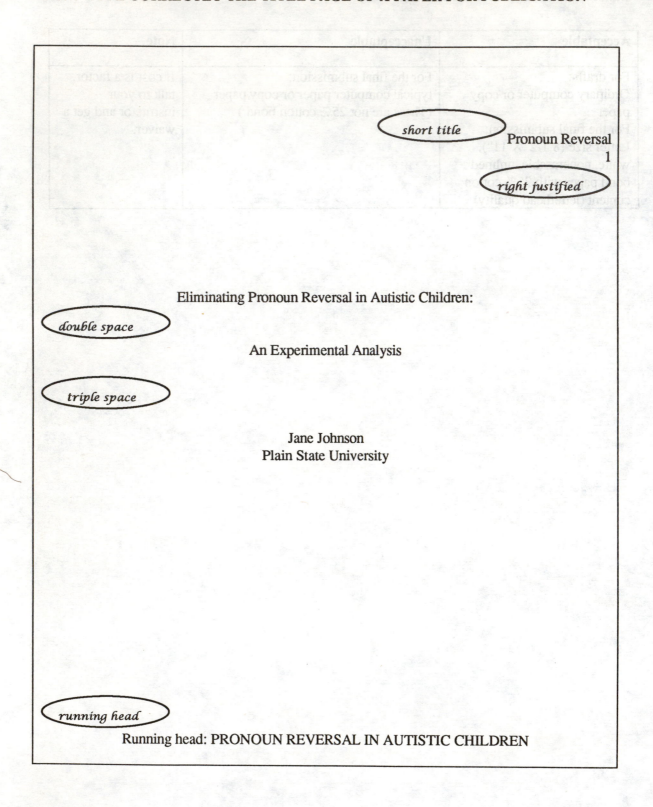

short title

Pronoun Reversal
1

right justified

Eliminating Pronoun Reversal in Autistic Children:

double space

An Experimental Analysis

triple space

Jane Johnson
Plain State University

running head

Running head: PRONOUN REVERSAL IN AUTISTIC CHILDREN

B.3.8. TYPE CORRECTLY THE TITLE PAGE OF A CLASS (TERM) PAPER

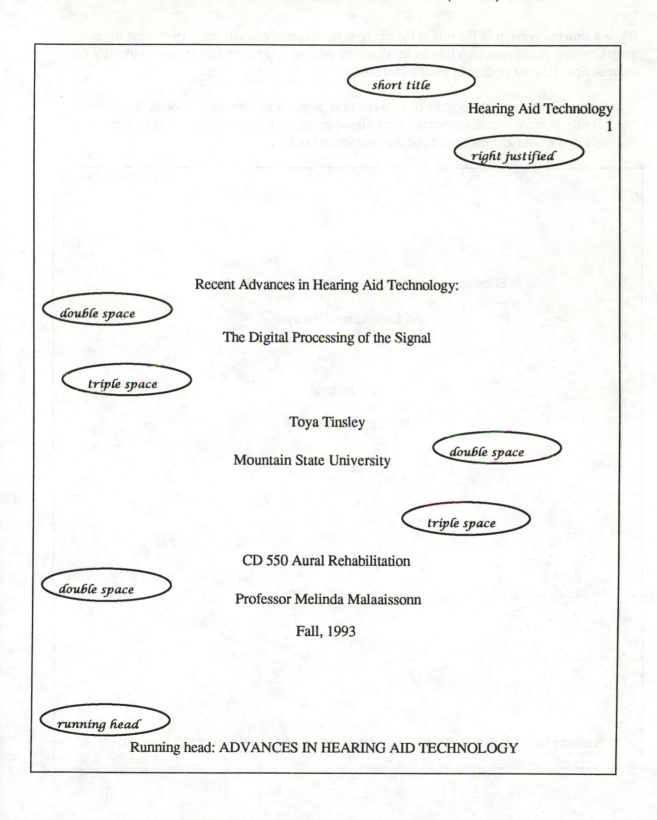

B3.9. TYPE THE SHORT TITLE AND THE RUNNING HEAD CORRECTLY

Type a **shorter version** of the title at the top right hand corner of **each page,** (including the title page), except pages on which figures are drawn or printed. This short title is only to identify the manuscript. It is not printed in a published article.

Type a **running head** at the bottom of **only the first page.** A running head, though shorter than the full title, is more complete than the short title at the top. The running head may be printed on the right or the left hand pages of published articles or books.

Pronoun Reversal
1

Eliminating Pronoun Reversal in Children with Autism:

An Experimental Analysis

Jane Johnson

Plain State University

Running head: ELIMINATING PRONOUN REVERSAL IN AUTISTIC CHILDREN

B.3.10. WRITE AN ABSTRACT ON THE SECOND PAGE

Type an abstract on the second page.

Type the word Abstract at the top, center portion of the page.

Do not indent the first line.

The short title and the page number appear on the top right-hand corner.

Double space the abstract.

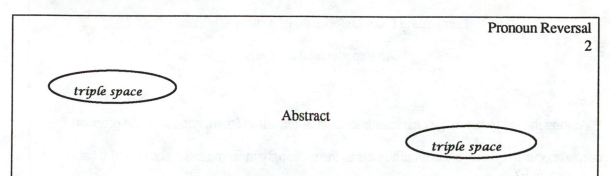

Pronoun reversal, a persistent language problem of children with autism has been difficult to eliminate. It has been suggested that echolalia, which is frequently observed in children with autism, may contribute to pronoun reversal. I tested this possibility by reducing echolalia with a time-out contingency and by measuring the frequency of pronoun reversal. Four autistic children between five and seven years of age were the subjects. I used the multiple baseline design across the four subjects. As the experimental contingency of time-out decreased the frequency of echolalia, the frequency of pronoun reversal also decreased.

B.3.11. BEGIN THE TEXT ON PAGE THREE

Pronoun Reversal
3

Eliminating Pronoun Reversal in Autistic Children:

An Experimental Analysis

Among the many language characteristics of children with autism, echolalia and pronoun reversal occur frequently. **Echolalia** refers to the seemingly meaningless repetition of what is heard. **Pronoun reversal** refers to the frequent substitution of an appropriate personal pronoun with an inappropriate pronoun. For example, an autistic child may substitute *you* for *me* and vice versa (Johnson, 1993)....

(text continued)

Note: Defined terms may be underlined, italicized, or printed in bold type.

B.3.12. NUMBER THE PAGES CORRECTLY

Do	Do not	Note
place the page number on the top right-hand corner, one line below the short title.	number the pages that contain figures and figure captions.	On most word processing programs, use the *Header* command to automatically insert page numbers.
number all pages of the paper consecutively, including the title page, tables, and other end materials.		Format page numbers as a right-aligned paragrph to print them at the end of right margin.
insert unnumbered pages at the end of the paper following all numbered material.		
renumber or repaginate the entire paper when you delete or add pages.	Do not give a new identity to the inserted page (e.g., 32A, 59B).	

B.3.13. REPRINT THE PAGES WITH CORRECTIONS

Do	Do not	Note
reprint or retype the corrected pages.	use handwritten corrections on your paper.	Final submission should be free from distracting corrections.
	use correction paper or liquid.	

B.3.14. INDENTATION

Indent	Do not indent	Note

five spaces:
   the first line of each
   paragraph of the text
   level four headings
three spaces:
   the second line of each
   reference on the reference
   list
	abstracts
	block quotations
	level three headings
	titles of tables
	legends of figures
	the first line of each reference on the reference list
		Most headings and titles are **centered.**
		Unindented lines are typed *flush left*.

B.3.15. GIVE CORRECT SPACE AFTER PUNCTUATION

Correct	Note
	one space after
Speech, language, and hearing The clinician said: "Stop!" Pronoun Reversal: An experimental treatment San Diego: Singular Publishing Group Q. X. Zenkin	commas semicolons the colon within a title the colon placed after the city of a publisher in the reference list periods of the initials of names
	two spaces after
So it went. But the problem was ... This is the rule: two spaces following ... Penn, P. Z. (1993). *Nation of Children*. New York: Infancy Press.	a period at the end of sentences *most* colons (see the other options) periods within a reference citation
	no space after
The male to female ratio of 4:1 has been reported.	a colon in ratios

B.3.16. USE THE HEADINGS WITHIN THE TEXT CONSISTENTLY

Headings should be brief and direct.

APA style includes up to five levels of headings.

Use the selected levels of headings consistently.

An introduction is untitled. (Do not type *Introduction.)*

For a research proposal you might submit to complete a class requirement, two levels of headings are adequate. Use additional levels if necessary.

Journals that use the APA style are not entirely faithful to all aspects of the APA style, especially to the levels of headings. Therefore, if you are required to follow the APA style, see the APA *Manual* for examples.

TWO LEVELS OF HEADINGS

Method ❶

(Centered Uppercase and Lowercase Heading)

<u>Subjects</u> ❷

(Flush Left, Underlined or Italicized, Uppercase and Lowercase Side Heading)

AN EXAMPLE OF TWO LEVELS OF HEADINGS

Hearing Impairment
8

(After an untitled introduction to the proposal, the following headings may be used.)

Method   ❶

Subjects ❷

 I will select 20 children from a special class for the hearing impaired. The children will come from middle–class families. The parents will have normal hearing ...

Procedure ❷

 The aural rehabilitation program to be evaluated will include an initial hearing evaluation, selecting and fitting of a hearing aid, parent counseling ...

Results   ❶

The results of the study are presented in Table 1. As the table shows, ...

Discussion   ❶

 Though many aural rehabilitation programs exist, few have been experimentally evaluated for their effectiveness. The present study shows that ...

A COMMON VARIATION OF TWO LEVELS OF HEADINGS

METHOD ❶

Subjects ❷

Materials ❷

Procedures ❷

RESULTS ❶

DISCUSSION ❶

Note that in this variation, the first level heading is typed in **all capitals.** Many journals use this format. The journals ASHA publishes show other variations in the way the articles are set up. Compare some of these variations with the APA style.

THREE LEVELS OF HEADINGS

Method ❶

(Centered Uppercase and Lowercase Heading)

<u>Procedure</u> ❷

(Flush Left, Underlined or Italicized, Uppercase and Lowercase Side Heading)

❸   <u>Baselines.</u> We established the baselines with 20 stimulus items. We used a series of modeled trials and a series of evoked trials ...

(Indented, underlined or italicized, lowercase paragraph heading ending with a period.
After two spaces, the text is started on the same line, as typed above.)

FOUR LEVELS OF HEADINGS

Experiment 2 ❶

(Centered Uppercase and Lowercase Heading)

<u>Method</u> ❷

(Centered, Underlined, Uppercase and Lowercase Heading)

<u>Materials</u> ❸

(Flush Left, Underlined or Italicized, Uppercase and Lowercase Side Heading)

❹ <u>Training pictures.</u> I will prepare the training pictures that represent ...

(Indented, underlined, lowercase paragraph heading ending with a period. After two spaces, the text is started on the same line, as typed above.)

FIVE LEVELS OF HEADINGS

EXPERIMENT 1: MORPHOLOGIC TRAINING ❶

(CENTERED UPPERCASE HEADING)

Establishing the Target Responses ❷

(Centered Uppercase and Lowercase Heading)

<u>Method</u> ❸

(Centered, Underlined, Uppercase and Lowercase Heading)

<u>Subjects</u> ❹

(Flush Left, Underlined or Italicized, Uppercase and Lowercase Side Heading)

❺   <u>The training procedure.</u> I used the incidental training procedure. In each session ...

  (Indented, underlined, lowercase paragraph heading ending with a period.
   After two spaces, the text is started on the same line, as typed above.)

B.3.17. WRITE OUT ABBREVIATIONS THE FIRST TIME YOU USE THEM AND ENCLOSE THE ABBREVIATION IN PARENTHESES

First Correct Citation	Subsequent Correct Citation	Note
The hearing threshold level (HTL) was measured ...	The HTL was ...	These audiological abbreviations need not be spelled out even the first time if an audiogram that spells them out accompanies the report or the reader is likely to know them.
A value of 100 Hertz (Hz) means that ...	A tone of 200 Hz was presented.	
A decibel (dB) is one tenth of a Bell.	In 5 dB increments ...	
The temporomandibular joint (TMJ) is an important joint ...	The TMJ is important for ...	
We measured the mean length of utterance (MLU) in syllables.	The obtained MLU values are shown in Table 1.	
The tone—a conditioned stimulus (CS)—may be presented ...	The intensity of CS was increased.	
You must obtain your Certificate of Clinical Competence (CCC).	The American Speech-Language-Hearing association issues the CCC in ...	
Our professional organization is the American Speech-Language Hearing Association (ASHA).	The president of ASHA spoke at the convention.	

B.3.18. DO NOT START A SENTENCE WITH A LOWER CASE ABBREVIATION

Incorrect	Correct	Note
dB is one tenth of a Bel.	The dB is one tenth of a Bel.	
ppb is useful in measuring the amount of pesticides in water.	The amount of the residual pesticide in water is measured in ppb.	These are the subsequent citations of the abbreviated words.

ppb = parts per billion

B.3.17. WRITE OUT ABBREVIATIONS THE FIRST TIME YOU USE THEM AND ENCLOSE THE ABBREVIATION IN PARENTHESES

Incorrect	Rewrite Correctly
The ASHA code of ethics is an important document. The members of ASHA should adhere to the code.	
In hearing evaluation, the SDT is a necessary measure to obtain. The (SDT) is the hearing level at which a person is just aware of speech.	
A loud noise is a UCS for startle response. The presentation of a UCS results in UCR.	
The LAD was proposed as the mechanism by which a young child derives the grammar of his or her language. Without the LAD, the child would be lost in confusion.	
In DLO, you specify the behavior that will not be reinforced. The effectiveness of DLO is well established.	
The child has a P.E. tube. Surgically implanted P.E. tubes allow for middle ear ventilation.	

ASHA: American Speech-Language-Hearing Association
SDT: Speech-detection threshold
UCS: Unconditioned stimulus; UCR: Unconditioned response
LAD: Language acquisition device
DLO: Differential reinforcement of other behavior
P.E. tube: Pressure-equalizing tube.

B.3.18. DO NOT START A SENTENCE WITH A LOWER CASE ABBREVIATION

Incorrect	Write Correctly
cc, being a metric measure ...	
lb is a popular measure in the U.S.	

cc: cubic centimeter   lb: pound

B.3.19. DO NOT WRITE OUT UNITS OF MEASUREMENT WHEN A NUMBER IS SPECIFIED

Incorrect	Correct	Note
20 seconds 2 hour 20 kilograms 5 centimeters 29 percent	20 sec 2 hr 20 kg 5 cm 29%	Abbreviated units of time are not written out in words; nor are units of measurement when accompanied by a number. They are always singular (e.g., kg, *not* kgs). Unless they are at the end of a sentence, there is no period at the end of these abbreviations. Exception: *in*. (for inch).

B.3.20. WRITE OUT UNITS OF MEASUREMENT WHEN A NUMBER IS NOT SPECIFIED

Incorrect	Correct	Note
The weight was specified in kg. (The specified weight was 10 kilograms.)	The weight was specified in kilograms. (The specified weight was 10 kg.)	
measured in cm ... (It was 10 centimeters long.)	measured in centimeters ... (It was 10 cm long.)	A specified number is always followed by an abbreviated unit of measure.
several lb of sugar (You have 10 pounds of sugar)	several pounds of sugar ... (You have 10 lb of sugar.)	
calculated the % of dysfluencies ... (The client had a 10 percent dysfluency rate.)	calculated the percentage of dysfluencies ... (The client had a 10% dysfluency rate.)	An unspecified unit of measure is always followed by a word, not an abbreviation.

B3.21. ADD THE PLURAL MORPHEME *S* TO PLURAL ABBREVIATIONS

(Do not add an apostrophe; add the *lower case* plural morpheme s)

Incorrect	Correct	Note
ABR's; ECG's; EEG's; IQ's; Ed's.; vol's.	ABRs; ECGs; EEGs; IQs; Eds.; vols.	A common mistake is to add an apostrophe

3.19.   DO NOT WRITE OUT UNITS OF MEASUREMENT WHEN A NUMBER IS SPECIFIED

Incorrect	Write Correctly
10 minute	
10 feet	
5 pounds	
Intelligence Quotient	

B.3.20.   WRITE OUT THE UNITS OF MEASUREMENT WHEN A NUMBER IS NOT SPECIFIED

Incorrect	Write Correctly
You can take several mg without side-effects.	
Stuttering persons' voice onset time was slower by several ms.	

mg: milligrams

ms: milliseconds

B3.21.   ADD THE PLURAL MORPHEME *S* TO PLURAL ABBREVIATIONS

Incorrect	Write Correctly
HTL's	
MLU's	
SRT's	
FR's	

B.3.22. WITH ABBREVIATIONS, USE THE PERIOD CORRECTLY

Add periods to	Do not add periods to
Initials of names (Z. Q. Xompompin)	Capital letter abbreviations and acronyms: ASHA; APA; UNESCO; PhD, IQ.
Geographic names (U.S. Military)	Abbreviations of state names: CA, NY
U.S. as an adjective (U.S. Department of Health and Human Services)	
Latin abbreviations: *i.e.; vs.; a.m.; e.g.*	
Reference abbreviations: *vol.; 2nd ed.; p.* 10.	

B.3.23. USE ROMAN NUMERALS ONLY WHEN IT IS AN ESTABLISHED PRACTICE

Incorrect	Correct
Cranial nerve 4	Cranial nerve IV
Type 2 error	Type II error

B.3.24. USE ARABIC NUMERALS FOR ALL NUMBERS LARGER THAN 10

Incorrect	Correct	Note
I selected eleven subjects.	I selected 11 subjects.	
The client is seventy-five years old.	The client is 75 years old.	Numbers 10 and above are not written in words unless they start a sentence.
The client met the training criterion on the fifteenth trial	The client met the training criterion on the 15th trial.	
The client was twenty percent dysfluent.	The client was 20% dysfluent.	

B.3.25. WRITE OUT IN WORDS NUMERALS BELOW 10

when they do not express precise measures
when they are not grouped for comparison with number 10 and above

Incorrect	Correct	Note
The client has missed 2 or 3 sessions this semester.	The client has missed two or three sessions this semester.	Precise measurement is not implied.
After 5 imitated responses, I will fade modeling.	After five imitated responses, I will fade modeling.	*Five* or *eight* is not in comparison with number 10 or above
I will use 8 items for training.	I will use eight items for training.	

B.3.22. WITH ABBREVIATIONS, USE THE PERIOD CORRECTLY

Incorrect	Write Correctly
US Park Service	
Secretary, US Department of Labor	
viz	
etc	

B.3.23. USE ROMAN NUMERALS ONLY WHEN IT IS AN ESTABLISHED PRACTICE

Incorrect	Write Correctly
Cranial nerve 8	
Type one error	

B.3.24. USE ARABIC NUMERALS FOR ALL NUMBERS LARGER THAN 10

Incorrect	Write Correctly
A caseload of fifty-five is large.	
The client met the training criterion in only twelve trials.	
The client's baserate production was fifteen percent.	

B.3.25. WRITE OUT IN WORDS NUMERALS BELOW 10

Incorrect	Write Correctly
At any one time, 4 to 5 students can observe the sessions.	
Approximately 7 weeks of training may be needed to meet the training criterion.	
My study will have 3 conditions.	
The client gave 7 responses.	

B3.26. WRITE OUT IN WORDS ANY NUMBER THAT BEGINS A SENTENCE

(Do not begin a sentence with a numeral.)

Correct	Incorrect	Note
5 children were tested.	Five children were tested.	No sentence is started with a number written in numerals.
7 clients attended all sessions and 4 did not attend any.	Seven clients attended all sessions and 4 did not attend any.	
75 clinicians attended the workshop.	Seventy-five clinicians attended the workshop.	
15% of the school children have some form of communicative disorders.	Fifteen percent of the school children have some form of communicative disorders.	

B.3.27. USE ARABIC NUMERALS WITH UNITS OF MEASUREMENT EVEN WHEN THE UNITS ARE BELOW TEN

(Still, of course, you cannot start a sentence with a numeral.)

Incorrect	Correct	Note
A five dB increment will be used.	A 5-dB increment will be used.	Though the numbers are below ten, they refer to specific units of measurement.
I will use a seven sec inter-trial interval.	I will use a 7-sec inter-trial interval.	

B.3.28. USE ARABIC NUMERALS WHEN NUMBERS BELOW 10 ARE COMPARED WITH NUMBERS 10 AND ABOVE

Incorrect	Correct	Note
The results show that seven of the 15 subjects improved.	The results show that 7 of the 15 subjects improved.	The smaller and the larger numbers are used in a comparative manner.
Modeling was used on the fourth and the 14th trials.	Modeling was used on the 4th and the 14th trials.	

B3.26. WRITE OUT IN WORDS ANY NUMBER THAT BEGINS A SENTENCE

Incorrect	Write Correctly
9 phonemes will be trained.	
39th percentile is not too impressive.	
37 children will be screened.	

B.3.27. USE ARABIC NUMERALS WITH UNITS OF MEASUREMENT EVEN WHEN THE UNITS ARE BELOW TEN

Incorrect	Write Correctly
A three-minute duration is too long for time-out.	
This is a seven lb bag.	

B.3.28. USE ARABIC NUMERALS WHEN NUMBERS BELOW 10 ARE COMPARED WITH NUMBERS 10 AND ABOVE

Incorrect	Write Correctly
The client did not respond on trials three and 12.	
Of the 15 subjects, the third and the 14th improved the most.	

B.3.29. DISTINGUISH BETWEEN A REFERENCE LIST AND A BIBLIOGRAPHY

A reference list lists the books, articles, and other sources cited in a piece of writing.

A bibliography is a list of all or most of the articles published on a topic.

A bibliography stands alone; it may not be attached to any text.

A reference list is always attached to a paper, a book, or other form of writing.

A reference list contains all that is cited and only what is cited in the text.

All scientific papers have reference citations in the text and a reference list at the end.

Term papers, theses, and other kinds of academic writing assignments also have reference citations in the text and a reference list at the end.

REFERENCE CITATION WITHIN THE TEXT

B3.30. CITE THE AUTHOR'S LAST NAME AND YEAR OF PUBLICATION IN THE TEXT

Incorrect	Correct	Note
In her study of heavyweight champions, Byson found that ...	In her study of heavyweight champions, Byson (1993) found that ...	The author's name is part of the narration. Therefore, only the year is in parentheses.
Ticklishson stated that humor is good medicine (1992).	Ticklishson (1992) stated that humor is good medicine.	Type the year immediately after the name.
Byson (1993) found that the reaction time of his opponents was sluggish.... Byson (1993) also found that ...	Byson (1993) found that the reaction time of his opponents was sluggish.... Byson also found that ...	Omit the year when the same study is referred to again within the same paragraph if it cannot be confused with another study.
A study showed that boxing causes brain damage; Hali, 1992.	A study showed that boxing causes brain damage (Hali, 1992).	When the name and the year are not a part of the narrative, enclose both within parentheses.
In (1978), MacVinro was the first to show that playing tennis sharpens the tongue.	In 1978, MacVinro was the first to show that playing tennis sharpens the tongue.	If the year also is a part of the narration, do not enclose it in parentheses.

B.3.31. CITE BOTH NAMES IN THE TEXT WHEN A WORK HAS TWO AUTHORS

Incorrect	Correct	Note
Tang et al., (1993) found that college courses are incomprehensible.	Tang and Lagassi (1993) found that college courses are incomprehensible.	Always, cite both the authors of a single work.

REFERENCE CITATION WITHIN THE TEXT

B.2.29. DISTINGUISH BETWEEN A REFERENCE LIST AND A BIBLIOGRAPHY

List the characteristics of a reference list and a bibliography

A reference list is:	A bibliography is:

B3.30. CITE THE AUTHOR'S LAST NAME AND YEAR OF PUBLICATION IN THE TEXT

Incorrect	Write Correctly
June Jinkson (1993) stated that ...	
In (1992), Torkinson reported that ...	
Jasperson's study has shown that ... (1992).	
It is known that bilingualism is enriching; Fung, 1992.	

B.3.31. CITE BOTH NAMES IN THE TEXT WHEN A WORK HAS TWO AUTHORS

Reference Information	Write a Sentence Using the Information
1. Authors: Cheng and Tang Year: 1993 Study on: Elimination of phonological processes Results: Only some processes were eliminated.	1. End the sentence with the reference:
2. Authors: Haniff and Chwe Year: 1992 Study on: incidence of stuttering in general population Result: about 1%.	2. Begin the sentence with the names:

B.3.32. CITE WORKS WITH THREE TO FIVE AUTHORS USING ALL THE AUTHORS' NAMES ONLY THE FIRST TIME

Subsequently, cite only the first author's last name and add "et al." to it. Include the year of publication.

Incorrect	Correct	Note
In a study on head injury, Hali, et al. (1993) found that ... *(first citation)*	In a study on head injury, Hali, Byson, and Tedson (1972) found that ... *(first citation)* The results of Hali et al. (1972) were that ... *(subsequent citation)*	Three authors, all cited the first time. *et al.* with no period after *et* (not *et. el.*); neither underlined nor italicized
In their study on vocal nodules, Lordon et al., (1992) discovered that ... *(first citation)* Lordon et al. (1989) showed that ... *(subsequent citation)*	In their study on vocal nodules, Lordon, Fontana, Tanseko, Pendl, and Tavratino (1992) discovered that ... *(first citation)* Lordon et al. (1989) showed that ... *(subsequent citation)*	Five authors, all cited the first time.

B3.33. CITE WORKS OF SIX OR MORE AUTHORS BY ONLY THE FIRST AUTHOR

Type "et al." after the first author's last name followed by the year of publication. Follow this rule even for the first citation.

Incorrect	Correct	Note
Wang, Bhat, Johnson, Hernadez, Allende, Singh, and Smith (1992) studied the effects of ... *(first citation)*	Wang et al. (1992) have studied the effects of ... *(first and subsequent citations).*	Add additional names only when it is necessary to distinguish works of multiple authors. See rule (B.3.32.).
Wren, Ram, Traveno, Kelly, Trudeau, and Boonthenthorpe (1993) reported that ... *(first citation)*	Wren et al. (1993) reported that ... *(first and subsequent citations).*	

B.3.32.   CITE WORKS WITH THREE TO FIVE AUTHORS USING ALL THE AUTHORS' NAMES ONLY THE FIRST TIME

Show both the **first** and one **subsequent** citations.

Reference Information	Write Sentences Using the Information
1. Authors: Shanker, Shantler, Samuelson, Whau, and Mistry Year: 1989 Study: New surgical methods of closing the complete palatal cleft Results: favorable 2. Authors: Southerland, Pena, and Pundit Year: 1990 Study: New methods of auditory masking Results: no improvement over existing methods	

B3.33.   CITE WORKS OF SIX OR MORE AUTHORS BY ONLY THE FIRST AUTHOR

Reference Information	Write a Sentence Using the Information
1. Authors: Soong, Moong, Moore, Raju, McLaughlin, and Johnson Year: 1993 Study on: noise suppression by digital hearing aids Results: very effective 2. Authors: Mann, Nath, Fahey, Lahey, Bohey, Johey, and Pinkerton Year: 1992 Study on: central auditory processing in stuttering persons Results: no abnormalities	

B.3.34. DISTINGUISH WORKS OF MULTIPLE AUTHORS PUBLISHED IN THE SAME YEAR

If two studies published in the same year with a different combination of three or more authors have the same first author:

cite all names if necessary;

or,

cite as many names as you need to distinguish the two studies.

Incorrect	Correct	Note
1. Lordon et al. (1992) showed that ... *(subsequent citation)* *(This study had four authors: Lordon, Fontana, Tanseko, and Pendl)* Lordon et al. (1992) have reported that ... *(subsequent citation)* *(A different study published in the same year that had a different combination of four authors: Lordon, Fontana, Tonseko, and Jensen)*	1. Lordon, Fontana, Tanseko, and Pendl (1992) showed that ... Lordon, Fontana, Tanseko, and Pendl (1992) also have reported that ... *(all names cited each time)* Lordon, Fontana, Tonseko, and Jensen (1992) have not shown a difference between the groups.	1. Though both are subsequent citations, all authors are cited to distinguish the two studies. If not, the two studies would be confused as they both abbreviate to Lordon et al. (1992).
2. Tinsonn et al. (1989) have found no significant difference. *(This study had seven authors: Tinsonn, Fung, Haniff, Chwe, Boonthenthorpe, Alvarado, and Smith)* Tinsonn et al. (1989) did not find the method effective. *(This study had six authors: Tinsonn, Fung, Mendoza, Kumar, Azevedo, and Alfonso)*	2. Tinsonn, Fung, et al. (1989) have found no significant difference. Tinsonn, Fung, Mendoza et al. (1989) did not find the method effective.	The two studies had six or more authors, published in the same year. Additional names distinguish the two studies.

B.3.34. DISTINGUISH WORKS OF MULTIPLE AUTHORS PUBLISHED IN THE SAME YEAR

Reference Information	Write a Sentence Using the Information
1. Authors: Rodriguez, Ford, Williams, and Benson Year: 1992 Study: effects of modeling on autistic children's speech Result: modeling increased children's echolalia 2. Authors: Rodriguez, Ford, Williams, Bennet, Bickley, Shekar, and Shinson Year: 1992 Study: assessment of language problems of children with mental retardation Results: numerous pragmatic problems	

B.3.35.   JOIN MULTIPLE NAMES WITH *AND* OR &

Join the names with *and* when the citation is part of the narrative.
Join the names with & (ampersand) when the citation is in parentheses.

Incorrect	Correct	Note
The survey study of Hecker & Donnors (1992) showed that crashing into each other is a profitable sport.	The survey study of Hecker and Donnors (1992) showed that crashing into each other is a profitable sport.	The names are a part of the narrative. Hence, the conjunction *and* is used.
It has been shown that the frequency of spitting on the field is related to the number of hits (Rosen and Tanseko, 1988).	It has been shown that the frequency of spitting on the field is related to the number of hits (Rosen & Tanseko, 1988).	The names are in parentheses. Hence, the ampersand is used.

B.3.36.   CITE MULTIPLE AUTHORS WITH THE SAME LAST NAME WITH THEIR INITIALS EVERY TIME THEY ARE CITED

Follow this rule even if the years are different.

Incorrect	Correct	Note
Connors (1992) and Connors (1968) reported that ... As discussed by Z. X. Connors et al. (1992) and Q. X. Connors (1992) ...	Z. X. Connors (1992) and Q. X. Connors (1993) reported that ... As discussed by Z. X. Connors et al. (1992) and Q. X. Connors (1992) ...	Connors (1992) and Connors (1993) refer to different studies, done by different authors.

B.3.35. JOIN MULTIPLE NAMES WITH *AND* OR &

Reference Information	Write a Sentence Using the Information
1. Part of narration Authors: Gimmick and Himmick Year: 1993 Study: the relation between screaming and vocal nodules Results: positive relation 2. Citation in parenthesis Authors: Byson and Lyson Year: 1992 Study: programming maintenance Results: possible to program maintenance	

B.3.36. CITE MULTIPLE AUTHORS WITH THE SAME LAST NAME WITH THEIR INITIALS EVERY TIME THEY ARE CITED

Reference Information	Write a Sentence Using the Information
Authors: B. D. Quayle (1992) and Z. Q. Quayle (1993) Study: variations in spelling the same word Results: discovered a variety of ways to spell the same word	
Authors: A. B. Perot et al. (1991) and B. C. Perot (1992) Study: how to reduce budget deficits Results: no way	

B.3.37. CITE MULTIPLE WORKS OF THE SAME AUTHOR IN A TEMPORALLY ASCENDING ORDER

Though you type multiple years, **do not** use the conjunction *and* before the final year (1989, 1990, 1992; but **not,** 1989, 1990, *and* 1992).

Incorrect	Correct	Note
Studies show that the more exciting the game, the greater the injury to vocal cords (Fontana, 1987, in press, 1992, 1990).	Studies show that the more exciting the game, the greater the injury to vocal cords (Fontana 1987, 1990, 1992, in press).	The *in press* citation is always the most recent.
Studies of Tonsiko and Travlatinova (1992, 1989, 1987, 1986) have shown that verbal abuse is a common locker room strategy.	Studies of Tonsiko and Travlatinova (1986, 1987, 1989, 1992) have shown that verbal abuse is a common locker room strategy.	The incorrect version is in the descending temporal order of publication.
Data suggest that the yells that induce vocal nodules excite the players (Rosery & Ruthery, 1981; 1978; 1975).	Data suggest that the yells that induce vocal nodules excite the players (Rosery & Ruthery, 1975, 1978, 1981).	Reference in parenthesis with the correct ascending order.

B.3.38. ATTACH ALPHABETICAL SUFFIXES TO THE SAME AUTHOR'S MULTIPLE PUBLICATIONS IN THE SAME YEAR

Repeat the year, do not affix a, b, c, and so forth to year typed only once (1989a, 1989b, 1989c; but **not** 1989a, b, c).

In assigning a, b, c, and so forth to studies published in the same year, use the alphabetical order of the first word of title of articles.

Incorrect	Correct	Note
Several studies by Johnson (1975-1, 1975-2, 1975-3, in press-1, in press-2) have shown that ...	Several studies (Johnson, 1975a, 1975b, 1975c, in press—a, in press—b) have shown that ...	Multiple *in press* entries also take a, b, c, and so forth.
Studies have shown that ball game watching increases brain size (Tonseko, 1985-1, 1985-2, 1985-3; 1988-1; 1988-2; Fontana, 1988-1, 1988-2; 1999-1, 1999-2; in press-1, in press-2).	Studies have shown that ball game watching increases brain size (Tonseko, 1985a, 1985b, 1985c; 1988a, 1988b; Fontana, 1988a, 1988b; 1999a, 1999b; in press—a, in press—b).	Multiple authors, each publishing multiple studies in two years; references in parentheses.

B.3.37. CITE MULTIPLE WORKS OF THE SAME AUTHOR IN A TEMPORALLY ASCENDING ORDER

Reference Information	Write a Sentence Using the Information
Author: McVinro Studies on: treatment of hoarse voice Studies published in: 1982, 1992, 1991, 1989	Include the author's name in your narration.
Author: Moncure and Sincure Studies on: bilingual-bicultural issues Studies published in: 1993, 1986, 1989, 1991	Enclose the authors' names in parentheses.
Author: Foresight Studies on: Future professional issues Studies published in: 1986, 1993, 1992, 1989, 1987.	Enclose the author's name in parentheses.

B.3.38. ATTACH ALPHABETICAL SUFFIXES TO THE SAME AUTHOR'S MULTIPLE PUBLICATIONS IN THE SAME YEAR

Reference Information	Write a Sentence Using the Information
Author: Sharp Studies: advances in cochlear implants Published: four in 1982.	Write the author's name as part of your narration.
Author: Bulltit Studies: dysphagia assessment techniques Published: three in 1992, two in 1993 Author: Hiltit Studies: dysphagia assessment techniques Published: two in 1989; two in 1992.	Cite the two authors and their publications in parentheses.

B.3.39. WITHIN PARENTHESES, ARRANGE THE LAST NAMES OF MULTIPLE AUTHORS IN ALPHABETICAL ORDER

Use the last name of the first author to determine the alphabetical order.
Separate each name with a semicolon.
Do not type *and* or *&* before the last citation

Incorrect	Correct	Note
(Zoom, 1990; Began, 1989; Push, 1985; Lord, 1980)	(Began, 1989; Lord, 1980; Push, 1985; Zoom, 1990)	Follow the alphabetical, not temporal, order.
(Push & Twink, 1991; Began & Quinn, 1980; Lord, Horde, & Board, 1975).	(Began & Quinn, 1980; Lord, Horde, & Board, 1975; Push & Twink, 1991).	The last name of the first author of a study determines the alphabetical order. The names of multiple authors are joined by an ampersand.
(Benson, 1989; Dinson, 1992; Henson, 1990; Nelson, 1986; and, Olsen, 1980).	(Benson, 1989; Dinson, 1992; Henson, 1990; Nelson, 1986; Olsen, 1980).	No *and* before the last entry.
(Bloodstein, 1967; Epstein, 1975; Fonstein, 1990; & Konstein, 1993)	(Bloodstein, 1967; Epstein, 1975; Fonstein, 1990; Konstein, 1993)	No ampersand before the last entry.

B.3.39. WITHIN PARENTHESES, ARRANGE THE LAST NAMES OF MULTIPLE AUTHORS IN ALPHABETICAL ORDER

Reference Information	Cite the Names Within Parentheses
1. Authors: Thompson, 1992 Johnson, 1993 Able, 1975 Quinn, 1993	
2. Authors: Zonks and Gonks, 1993 Banks and Atkins, 1990 Atkins, 1960 Kinson, 1992	

REFERENCE LIST

B.3.40. BEGIN THE REFERENCE LIST ON A NEW PAGE WITH A CENTERED, UPPERCASE, AND LOWERCASE HEADING

Double space the entire Reference List.

Pronoun Reversal
21

References

Able, T. K. (1989). *The autistic children.* New York: Sapson Press.

Babble, B. B. (1993). The negative effects of modeling on echolalia. *Journal of Autism,*

   10, 19-25.

Sunson, K. J. (1992). Foundations of educational research. Bend, IN: Prince Publishing.

Zonks, Z. Z. (1976). *Treatment of autistic children.* San Francisco: Zing Press.

REFERENCE LIST

B.3.40. BEGIN THE REFERENCE LIST ON A NEW PAGE WITH A CENTERED, UPPERCASE, AND LOWERCASE HEADING

Write a running head, an arbitrarily selected page number, and the word *references* with the right characters and in the correct position.

B.3.41. IN THE REFERENCE LIST, ARRANGE REFERENCES IN ALPHABETICAL ORDER

Use the last name to determine the alphabetical order.

Alphabetize the names of multiple authors by the surname of the first author.

Alphabetize names letter by letter, but exclude the initials.

Arrange prefixes in their strict alphabetical order. Ignore an apostrophe attached to a prefix (M').

Consult the biographical section of *Webster's New Collegiate Dictionary* to find the order in which surnames with articles and prepositions are arranged (names with de, la, du, von, etc.).

When listing several works by the same author, but some with and some without co-authors, start with those works that do not have co-authors

Incorrect	Correct	Note
McNeil Macmillan	Macmillan McNeil	*Mac* precedes *Mc*
Thomson, A. B. Thomas, Z. X.	Thomas, Z. X. Thomson, A. B.	Alphabetized letter-by-letter. The initials are ignored.
Tonseko, K. J., & Fontana, P. J. (1982) Tonseko, K. J., & Lordon, T. P. (1984) Tonseko, K. J. (1988) Tonseko, K. J. (1985)	Tonseko, K. J. (1985) Tonseko, K. J. (1988) Tonseko, K. J., & Fontana, P. J. (1982) Tonseko, K. J., & Lordon, T. P. (1984)	Single author entered first. Second authors are alphabetized, too: *Tonseko & Fontana* before *Tonseko & Lordon*

B.3.42. ARRANGE MULTIPLE WORKS OF THE SAME SINGLE AUTHOR FROM THE EARLIEST TO THE LATEST YEAR

Incorrect	Correct	Note
Able, P. J. (1993) Able, P. J. (1992) Able, P. J. (1989)	Able, P. J. (1989) Able, P. J. (1992) Able, P. J. (1993)	For each single author, the arrangement is from the earliest to the latest year.
Benson, L. S. (1992) Benson, L. S. (1982) Benson, L. S. (1972)	Benson, L. S. (1972) Benson, L. S. (1982) Benson, L. S. (1992)	

B.3.41. IN THE REFERENCE LIST, ARRANGE REFERENCES IN ALPHABETICAL ORDER

Reference Information	Arrange the Names Alphabetically
McMinnan McDonald McFarrin Van Riper Axelrod Herbert Hernadez Alvarado von Kirk de Klerk	

B.3.42. ARRANGE MULTIPLE WORKS OF THE SAME SINGLE AUTHOR FROM THE EARLIEST TO THE LATEST YEAR

Reference Information	Arrange the Names in the Correct Order
Larson, K. (1988) Larson, K. (1986) Larson, K. (1980)	
McDonald, P. (1993) McDonald, P. (1975) McDonald, P. (1974)	

B.3.43. ALPHABETIZE THE TITLES OF SEVERAL WORKS OF THE SAME AUTHOR PUBLISHED IN THE SAME YEAR

Ignore such words as *A* and *The* at the beginning of the title.
Attach the lowercase letters a, b, c, and so forth to the year of publication.

Incorrect	Correct	Note
Lagassi, A.R. (1991a). Problems of clay courts Lagassi, A. R. (1991b). Advantages of short-handled rackets.	Lagassi, A. R. (1991a). Advantages of short-handled rackets. Lagassi, A.R. (1991b). Problems of clay courts.	The first words of the title determine the order: *Advantages* precedes *Problems*.
Massood, P. T. (1992a). Some advantages of the circular paper clips. Massood, P. T. (1992b). The case of the missing paper clip.	Massood, P. T. (1992a). The case of the missing paper clip. Massood, P. T. (1992b). Some advantages of the circular paper clips.	The article *The* is ignored in arranging these two entries.

B.3.44. ALPHABETIZE THE DIFFERENT AUTHORS OF THE SAME LAST NAME ACCORDING TO THEIR INITIALS

Incorrect	Correct	Note
Able, Q. T. (1993) Able, A. A. (1982)	Able, A. A. (1982) Able, Q. T. (1993)	The year of publication does not matter
Tavratinova, S. N. (1987) Tavratinova, B. D. (1993)	Tavratinova, B.D. (1987) Tavratinova, S.N. (1993)	

B.3.43. ALPHABETIZE THE TITLES OF SEVERAL WORKS OF THE SAME AUTHOR PUBLISHED IN THE SAME YEAR

Reference Information	Alphabetize According to the Titles
Belwae, T. P. (1989a). A potential explanation of muddy football fields. Belwae, T. P. (1989b). Crashing and winning: The cultural underpinnings of football.	
Cisnero, S. M. (1990a). Cities in decay. Cisnero, S. M. (1990b). Banking on the neighborhood.	

B.3.44. ALPHABETIZE THE DIFFERENT AUTHORS OF THE SAME LAST NAME ACCORDING TO THEIR INITIALS

Reference Information	Alphabetize According to the Initials
Nelson, Z. T. (1988) Nelson, B. S. (1990) Nelson, A. P. (1986)	
Ramig, L. T. (1993) Ramig, C. C. (1990) Ramig, B. D. (1991)	

B.3.45.   TYPE FLUSH LEFT THE FIRST LINE OF EACH ENTRY AND INDENT THE SECOND AND SUBSEQUENT LINES THREE SPACES

Incorrect	Correct	Note
Lagassi, A. R. (1991a). Problems of clay courts Lagassi, A. R. (1991b). Advantages of short-handled rackets.	Lagassi, A. R. (1991a). Advantages of short-handled rackets. Lagassi, A.R. (1991b). Problems of clay courts.	The first line is not indented (flush left).
Massood, P. T. (1992a). Some advantages of the circular paper clips. Massood, P. T. (1992b). The case of the missing paper clip.	Massood, P. T. (1992a). The case of the missing paper clip. Massood, P. T. (1992b). Some advantages of the circular paper clips.	Second and subsequent lines are indented three spaces.

B.3.46.   USE THE FOLLOWING ABBREVIATIONS IN THE REFERENCE LISTS

Abbreviation	For	Note
chap.	chapter	Lowercase abbreviations.
ed.	edition	
rev. ed.	revised edition	
2nd ed.	second edition	
Ed. (Eds.)	Editor (Editors)	(Eds.) period within the closing parenthesis.
Trans.	Translator(s)	The same abbreviation for the singular or plural.
p. (pp.)	page (pages)	Lowercase.
Vol.	Volume	Uppercase; as in Vol. 7 of a journal or book.
vols.	volumes	Lowercase for the plural *volumes*.
No.	Number	Uppercase; do not type # for number.
Pt.	Part	Uppercase.
Tech. Rep.	Technical Report	Both the abbreviated words in uppercase.
Suppl.	Supplement	Uppercase.

B.3.45. TYPE FLUSH LEFT THE FIRST LINE OF EACH ENTRY AND INDENT THE SECOND AND SUBSEQUENT LINES BY THREE SPACES

Incorrect	Rewrite Correctly
Sherma, P. K. (1989). The influence of the mother's vocabulary on the child's language acquisition. Tackle, K. K. (1990). Tackle football and the moral fiber.	

B.3.46. USE THE FOLLOWING ABBREVIATIONS IN THE REFERENCE LISTS

Unabbreviated	Write the Correct Abbreviation
chapter	
edition	
revised edition	
second edition	
Editor (Editors)	
Translator(s)	
page (pages)	
Volume	
volumes	
Number	
Part	
Technical Report	
Supplement	

SELECTED EXAMPLES OF REFERENCES

See The APA *Manual* (1983) for other examples.

B.3.47. JOURNAL ARTICLES

- Give one space after the last initial. Type a period after the year in parentheses. Give two spaces before starting the article title.
- Type a coma after the last initial of the first author and join the names of two authors with an ampersand (&).
- Give two spaces before the journal name is typed.
- Capitalize all important words of the journal name; do not abbreviate journal titles; and underline or italicize the entire title.
- Underline or italicize the volume number, but do not type the word *volume* or its abbreviation.
- Enter the page number or numbers as the last entry without *p.* or *pp*.
- For an article in press, do not give date, volume number, or page number. Replace the year of publication with the words "in press."
- Indent three spaces from the left–hand margin the second and subsequent lines of each reference.

Correct	Note
Bultit, B. S., Airhead, E. H., & Longwind, H. A. (1990). Intervening variables in human behavior: Thirty years of theorizing. *Journal of Theories Unlimited, 98,* 3-78.	A comma and a space separate each name.
Hazelnut, L. M., & Beachnut P. M. (in press). Nutty theories in naughty disciplines. *Journal of Speculative Psychology.*	A coma precedes an ampersand.
Lordon, M. S. (1987). The offensive tactics on the football field and delayed aphasic symptoms. *Journal of Speech and Hearing Disorders, 42,* 50-58.	Two spaces separate the year and the article title. The journal title and the volume number are italicized (or underline).
McVenro, J. P. (1990). The relation between umpire judgments and player verbal outbursts. *Journal of Verbal Abuse, 50,* 230-240.	

SELECTED EXAMPLES OF REFERENCES

B.3.47. JOURNAL ARTICLES

Reference Information	Correctly Write the References
Author: P. T. Lang Year 1992 Article Title: The grammar of American Sign Language. Journal: Journal of Nonverbal Communication. Volume: 10 Pages: 15-25.	
Author: S. L. Nunez Year: in press Article Title: Models of counseling in speech and hearing. Journal: American Journal of Speech-Language Pathology.	
Authors: K. K. Rimm and B. B. Brimm Year: 1989 Article Title: The relation between maternal intonation and the child's singing ability Journal: Journal of Music Therapy Volume: 12 Pages: 13-23	

B.3.48. BOOKS

- Underline or italicize the title of the book. Capitalize only the first letter of the title and subtitle.
- Give two spaces between the year and the title, and between the title and the place of publication.
- Type the abbreviated word *Jr.* after the last initial, if applicable.
- Type the abbreviated edition number (2nd ed.) or the words "rev. ed." (for revised edition) after the title and place within parentheses.
- Type the name of the city of the publisher.
- If the city is not well–known or could be confused with another location, type the abbreviated name of the state. Use the U.S. Postal Service abbreviations for the states.
- Type the publishing company's name exactly as it appears in the book being referenced.
- For books written and published by corporations, agencies, or associations, type the word "Author" for the publisher.

Correct	Note
American Psychological Association. (1983). *Publication manual of the American Psychological Association* (3rd ed.). Washington, DC: Author.	The publisher and the author are the same (a corporate author). *DC* is added to Washington because it could be confused with the state of Washington.
Boczquats, N. S. (1990). *Oceanography and communication: A new frontier*. Chicago: Blue Heaven Press.	Two spaces separate: the year and the title; the title and the place of publication.
Histrionik, K. L., Jr., & Stoic, P. L. (1975). *Neurotic behavior* (2nd ed.). Los Angeles: Angeles Publishing Company.	The book edition in parentheses; not italicized.
Null, B. D. (1988). *Numbers in civilization* (rev. ed.). New York: Sappleton.	(rev. ed.) for revised edition.
Blinton, W., & Blinton, H. (1993). *Hope for America*. Hope, AR: Optimist Press.	The state abbreviation is added because the city is not well–known. A colon—not a period— follows the state abbreviation.

B.3.48. BOOKS

Reference Information	Correctly Write the References
Author: K. D. Wong Title: Bilingual Speech-Language Pathology Year: 1993 Edition: Second Publisher: Word Publishing Company City: Ames, Iowa	
Authors: S. S. Simms, T. T. Tinns, and K. K. Kimms Title: Education of Children with Central Auditory Problems Edition: Revised Year: 1990 Publisher: Nelson Publishers City: New York, New York	
Author: N. C. Gordimeir Title: Hearing Aids of the Future Year: 1929 Publisher: The Future Press City: Hazletown, Tennessee	
Author: American Speech-Language-Hearing Association Title: Your Professional Organization Year: 1988 City: Rockville Pike, Maryland Publisher: American Speech-Language-Hearing Association	

B.3.49. EDITED BOOKS AND CHAPTERS IN EDITED BOOKS

- Type in parentheses the abbreviated word (Ed.) for one editor or (Eds.) for multiple editors.
- Type (ed.) for an edition of a book.
- Place the author's initials at the end of the surname *(as usual)*.
- Place the editor's initials at the beginning, not the end of the surname *(not as usual)*.
- Type the pages of the chapter after the title and within parentheses.

Correct	Note
Baker, K. V. (1986). The unknown and the unconscious. In C. Hart (Ed.), *Unknown and inaccessible states of consciousness* (pp. 305-395). New York: Mystery Publishing House.	In the text, the author of the chapter, not the editor of the book, is cited (Baker, 1986, not Hart, 1986). Author's initials and the editor's initials are in reversed positions. The page numbers are for the cited author's chapter only.
Hunt, C. P., & Holms, G. S. (Eds.). (1980). *Mysteries of mental events*. Clovis, CA: Invisible Publishers.	This reference is for an entire edited book. (Eds.) for Editors
Xong, K. C. (Ed.). (1990). *Split brain is just as good*. Los Angeles: NeuroPress.	(Ed.) for Editor

B.3.50. REPORTS FROM ORGANIZATIONS AND GOVERNMENT AGENCIES

Correct	Note
National Child Health and Human Development. (1910). How not to write research proposals (DHHS Publication No. QRS-00910). Washington, DC: U.S. Government Printing Office.	"Publication No," "Report No," and so forth are in parentheses;
Norm, J. J. (1989). *Invariably fixed stages of cognitive development* (Report No. 15). Washington, DC: National Cognition Association.	The period is typed after the closing parenthesis; no period is typed at the end of the actual title of the report.

B.3.49. EDITED BOOKS AND CHAPTERS IN EDITED BOOKS

Reference Information	Correctly Write the References
Editors: L. B. Johns and R. K. Bangs Title: Professional Issues in Speech-Language Pathology Year: 1992 Publisher: College Press City: Los Angeles	
Author: N. O. Jackson Chapter title: Speech-language pathologist and the bilingual child Year: 1993 Pages: 135-175 Book title: Education in the Next Century Editors: A.K. Cantor and B. L. Bantor Publisher: Century Press City: Portland, Oregon	

B.3.50. REPORTS FROM ORGANIZATIONS AND GOVERNMENT AGENCIES

Reference Information	Correctly Write the References
Organization: National Institute of Public Health (NIPH) Year: 1993 Title of Publication: Threats to Public Health Publication #PQ-01-S25 City: Washington, DC From: U. S. Government Printing Press	
Author: S. L. Beans Title: Brain and Behavior Year: 1990 Publisher: National Neuroscience Association Report #67 City: Baltimore, Maryland	

B.3.51. PROCEEDINGS OF CONFERENCES AND CONVENTIONS

Correct	Note
Peacock, P. L., & Lyon, A. D. (1990). Cooperation among the animal kingdoms of the world. In E. L. Phant & H. I. Pottoms (Eds.), *Proceedings of the Ninety Fourth International Symposium of the Animal Kingdom* (pp. 23-57). Boston: Cobra Press.	The title of the paper is not italicized, but the title of the proceedings published as a book is.

B.3.52. CONVENTION PRESENTATIONS

Correct	Note
Idlemann, P. S. (1983, November). *Variables related to doing nothing.* Paper presented at the Annual Meeting of the American Anti-workaholic Association, Bullhead City, AZ.	"Meeting," "convention," and so forth should be accurate. The title of presentation should be underlined or italicized.
Hernandez, K. S. (1992, November). *Caseload issues in public schools.* Paper presented at the Annual Convention of the American Speech-Language-Hearing Association, San Antonio, TX.	Give the month in parentheses. End with the name of the city and the state abbreviation.

B.3.53. UNPUBLISHED ARTICLES, THESES, OR DISSERTATIONS

Correct	Note
Dimm, B. J. (1975). *Why some articles do not get published.* Unpublished manuscript.	Titles are underlined or italicized.
Brightly, B. B. (1975). *The complex relationship between self-image, hair color, and academic learning in children from low, medium, and high income levels.* Unpublished master's thesis, Sharp College of Education, Needles, CA.	
Smiley, S. S. (1985). *Variables related to early or late toilet training and the frequency of smiling in high school classrooms.* Unpublished doctoral dissertation, Haywire University, Lynn, OH.	The name of the university, the city, and the state abbreviations end the citation

B.3.51. PROCEEDINGS OF CONFERENCES AND CONVENTIONS

Reference Information	Correctly Write the References
Author: D. V. Quietson Paper: Hearing impairment in rock musicians Pages: 87-97 Title of the book: Proceedings of the 10th national symposium on noise and hearing loss Editors of the book: C. D. Noysman and F. S. Loudman Year: 1990 City: Centralia, Illinois Publisher: Peace Press	

B.3.52. CONVENTION PRESENTATIONS

Reference Information	Correctly Write the References
Author: B. J. Beans Paper: A new method of scoring language samples Presented at: National Convention of the American Speech-Language-Hearing Association Date: November, 1990 City: Atlanta, Georgia	

B.3.53. UNPUBLISHED ARTICLES, THESES, OR DISSERTATIONS

Reference Information	Correctly Write the References
Author: T. K. Henkly Unpublished Article: How to get published in speech and hearing	
Author: G. V. Gyon M.A. thesis: Evaluation of an early language intervention package Year,: 1990 University: Downstate University City: Rocks, New Jersey	

WRITING THE DIFFERENT SECTIONS OF A PAPER

B.3.54. WRITE THE *REVIEW*, THE *METHODS*, AND THE *RESULTS* OF COMPLETED STUDIES IN THE PAST TENSE

Incorrect	Correct
Deegook (1985) reports similar findings	Deegook (1985) reported similar findings.
The author selects 10 male and 10 female subjects.	The author selected 10 male and 10 female subjects.
In assessing the hearing of the subjects, the Nicolet Aurora Model 1020 is used.	In assessing the hearing of the subjects, the Nicolet Aurora Model 1020 was used.
The results show that back massage is not effective in reducing stuttering.	The results showed that back massage was not effective in reducing stuttering.

B.3.55. WRITE THE *DISCUSSION* SECTION IN THE PRESENT TENSE

Only an already completed study will have a discussion section. Research proposals do not have a discussion section.

Incorrect	Correct
The data *suggested* that further research is needed.	The data *suggest* that further research is needed.
The results *implied* that damage to Broca's area is not necessary to produce Broca's aphasia.	The results *imply* that damage to Broca's area is not necessary to produce Broca's aphasia.

B.3.56. WRITE THE *REVIEW* SECTION OF A *RESEARCH PROPOSAL* IN THE PAST TENSE

Incorrect	Correct
The results of past studies show that patients with aphasia recover the most within the first 6 months of post-onset (Bikling, 1986; Thomas, 1992; Wise, 1988).	The results of past studies have shown that patients with aphasia recover the most within the first 6 months of post-onset (Bikling, 1986; Thomas, 1992; Wise).
Smith and Jones (1980) report that their test on central auditory processing is a useful diagnostic tool.	Smith and Jones (1980) reported that their test on central auditory processing is a useful diagnostic tool.

WRITING THE DIFFERENT SECTIONS OF A PAPER

B.3.54. WRITE THE *REVIEW* , THE *METHODS*, AND THE *RESULTS* OF COMPLETED STUDIES IN THE PAST TENSE

Incorrect	Write Correctly
Smith (1989) believes that the classification of aphasia is an unnecessary exercise.	
Johnson (1967) uses the interview method to gather information on stuttering onset.	
The results of the Hanson (1988) study show that conductive hearing impairment is common in children.	

B.3.55. WRITE THE *DISCUSSION* SECTION IN THE PRESENT TENSE

Incorrect	Correct
The meaning of these results was not clear.	
The findings did not support the theory of unconscious control of the speech mechanism.	

B.3.56. WRITE THE *REVIEW* SECTION OF A *RESEARCH PROPOSAL* IN THE PAST TENSE

Incorrect	Write Correctly
The result of the Smith and Jones (1993) study supports the use of phonological analysis.	
Several past studies document the effectiveness of a well designed aural rehabilitation program.	

B.3.57. WRITE THE *METHODS* AND *EXPECTED RESULTS* SECTIONS OF A *PROPOSAL* IN THE FUTURE TENSE

A proposal may have an **expected results** section in which the author describes the potential outcome of the proposed study.

Incorrect	Correct
I selected the subjects randomly.	I will select subjects randomly. The subjects will be selected randomly.
I used the ABAB single-subject design.	I will use the ABAB single-subject design. The ABAB single-subject design will be used.
The results supported my hypothesis.	I expect the results to support my hypothesis.

B.3.57. WRITE THE *METHODS* AND *EXPECTED RESULTS* SECTIONS OF A *PROPOSAL* IN THE FUTURE TENSE

Incorrect	Write Correctly
I used 20 hearing impaired subjects in the study.	
I modeled when the client did not respond to my questions.	
The results suggested that cochlear implants were effective.	

Note to Students Working on Theses or Dissertations

The graduate schools of most universities have a set of guidelines on the preparation of theses and dissertations. Even the departments of communicative disorders that accept the APA style may have special guidelines that deviate in certain respects from the APA style. Therefore, students should consult both the APA style and the guidelines of their department and the graduate school.

B.4. PARTS OF A RESEARCH PAPER

Printed Notes	Class Notes

Abstract

An abstract highlights the problems, the methods, the procedures, and the results of a scientific paper in direct and nonevaluative language. It is written not only to give a summary of the article, but also to attract the reader to the whole article. An abstract is printed on a separate page.

According to the APA *Manual* (1983), a good abstract is accurate, self-contained, concise and specific, nonevaluative, and coherent and readable. The *Manual* limits the abstract of a report to 100 to 150 words, and that of a review article to 75 to 100 words.

Introduction

The text of the paper starts with an introductory section without a heading. This section introduces: (1) the general area of investigation, (2) the general findings of past investigations, (3) the specific topic of the current investigation, (4) a review of selected studies that have dealt with the topic in the past, (5) the methods, results, conclusions, methodological problems, and limitations of the past studies, (6) the questions that remain to be answered, (7) the significance of the current investigation, and (8) the specific problem or research questions investigated in the present study.

| Printed Notes | Class Notes |

The introduction should move from the general topic of investigation to the particular, specific research question. The critical review of previous studies should be fair, objective, and direct. The review should make clear to the reader the need for the study and the reasoning behind it. The review should show how the present study is related to past research while also pointing out its innovative aspects. Toward the end of the introduction, the research question should be formally stated. Hypotheses, if proposed, may be stated at this point. The research questions and hypotheses must be written in direct, clear, and terse language. By giving a good background, an introduction sets the stage for the study.

METHOD

The second section describes the method in detail for two reasons: (1) to give sufficient information to the reader who can understand the methods and procedures of the study to judge their appropriateness to investigate the research questions asked and (2) to permit direct and systematic replications of the study.

The method section consists of at least three subsections: (1) the subjects, (2) the apparatus or materials, and (3) the procedure. Additional subsections, such as baselines or probe, may be necessary.

Do not confuse the *METHOD* with *Procedures*. **METHOD** is a first level heading and **Procedures** is a second level heading.

Printed Notes	Class Notes

Subjects

The relevant characteristics of the subject (gender, age, education, occupation, family background, health, geographical location, and communicative behaviors) are described. The number of subjects selected and subject selection procedure also are described in this subsection.

In clinical studies, the subjects' diseases and disorders should be described in both qualitative and quantitative terms. Generally, any subject characteristic thought to influence the results should be described.

Materials

This subsection describes the physical setting of the study and the names and model numbers of equipment used. Standardized or nonstandardized tests and other procedures are summarized. Photographs, diagrams, or additional descriptions can be included in an appendix if the apparatus is unusual or rarely used.

Procedures

This subsection describes in detail how the study was implemented. The experimental design should be identified and explained in greater detail if uncommon. The author should report all stimuli presented to the subjects, how variables were measured and manipulated, and the temporal sequence of various conditions arranged in the study.

Differences in the treatment of groups of subjects should be explained, as well as reliability of the data. In reporting clinical treatment studies, the author should describe in detail the treatment procedures and how they were implemented. The methods by which the treatment effects were measured and evaluated also should be described.

Other procedural information may be included in this section. In making this section complete, the author should follow the rule of providing all information necessary to replicate the study.

RESULTS

The results section opens with a brief statement of the problem investigated and the general findings of the study. An overview of the results is followed by a detailed presentation of quantitative, qualitative, graphic, and tabular presentation of the findings. These findings are reported without evaluations and interpretations.

Tables and graphs may be used to display data. Tables and graphs should supplement, not duplicate the text. Statistical or other procedures of data analysis should be specified and, when necessary, justified.

In organizing the results of a study, the student must consult the APA *Manual* and several exemplary articles published in the professional journal to which the author plans to submit the paper for publication.

Printed Notes	Class Notes

DISCUSSION

In the discussion section, the author points out the meaning and significance of the results. After opening with a brief statement of the problem and results, the section discusses the theoretical and applied implications of the findings. The results are related to findings from previous investigations.

Limitations of the study also are pointed out, along with suggestions for further research. Ideally, a discussion is an integrative essay on the topic investigated, but it is written in light of the data generated by the study. It should answer research questions posed in the introduction, as well as support or refute any hypotheses presented. Clarity and directness are important here. Excessive speculation on the causes of unexpected data should be avoided.

REFERENCES

The references list publications and other sources of information cited in the paper. The reference list should be accurate. It should be prepared according to an accepted format, such as that of the APA *Manual*. It should list all of, and only, the sources cited in the paper.

Note to Students on Different Formats of Journal Articles

Besides research papers (articles), scientific and professional journals publish review papers, theoretical papers, tutorials, commentaries, and other kinds of papers. Each type of paper has an accepted format. Students should consult journals of their discipline and study types of papers and their prescribed formats.

PART C

PROFESSIONAL WRITING

Note to Student Clinicians

Professional writing includes writing diagnostic or assessment reports, treatment plans, progress reports, and professional correspondence. On the following pages, you will find examples and variations of each of these types of reports. Study them carefully and compare them with those written in your clinic.

C.1. DIAGNOSTIC REPORTS

Diagnostic reports also may be known as assessment reports and evaluation reports. In this book, the terms *diagnostic reports, assessment reports,* and *evaluation reports* are used interchangeably.

ELEMENTS OF A DIAGNOSTIC REPORT

Although the formats vary, all diagnostic reports contain the following kinds of information:

- History of the client, the family, and the disorder
- Interview of the family, the client, or both
- Orofacial examination
- Hearing screening
- Speech and language samples
- Disorder-specific assessment
- Diagnostic summary
- Recommendations

On the following pages, you will see outlines of typical diagnostic or assessment reports. Note that:

- The various headings and subheadings may vary across clinics and clinicians
- Most clinicians include information of the kind the headings suggest
- All headings and subheadings are not needed for all clients

---

C.1.1. OUTLINE OF A TYPICAL DIAGNOSTIC REPORT ON A *CHILD CLIENT*

UNIVERSITY SPEECH AND HEARING CLINIC

Victorville, California

DIAGNOSTIC REPORT

CLIENT: BIRTH DATE:

ADDRESS: CLINIC FILE NUMBER:

CITY: DATE OF REPORT:

TELEPHONE NUMBER: DIAGNOSIS:

REFERRED BY: CLINICIAN:

BACKGROUND AND REASONS FOR REFERRAL

HISTORY

Birth and Development

Medical History

Family, Social, and Educational History

ASSESSMENT INFORMATION

Orofacial Examination

Hearing Screening

Speech Production and Intelligibility

Language Production and Comprehension

Fluency

Voice

DIAGNOSTIC SUMMARY

RECOMMENDATIONS

Submitted by_____

    Thomas Jefferson, B.A.

    Student Clinician

Approved By_____

    Mary Lincoln, M.A., CCC-SP

    Speech-Language Pathologist and Clinical Supervisor

C.1.2. OUTLINE OF A TYPICAL DIAGNOSTIC REPORT ON AN *ADULT CLIENT*

**UNIVERSITY SPEECH AND HEARING CLINIC
JEFFERSON CITY, NORTH CAROLINA**

DIAGNOSTIC REPORT

CLIENT: BIRTH DATE:

ADDRESS: CLINIC FILE NUMBER:

CITY: DATE OF REPORT:

TELEPHONE NUMBER: DIAGNOSIS:

REFERRED BY: CLINICIAN:

BACKGROUND AND REASONS FOR REFERRAL

HISTORY

Medical History

Family and Social History

Educational and Occupational History

ASSESSMENT INFORMATION

Orofacial Examination

Hearing Screening

Speech Production and Intelligibility

Language Production and Comprehension

Fluency

Voice

DIAGNOSTIC SUMMARY

RECOMMENDATIONS

Submitted by_____

      June Ahmed, B.A.

      Student Clinician

Approved By_____

      April Summers, M.A., CCC-SP

      Speech-Language Pathologist and Clinical Supervisor

C.1.3. ANATOMY OF AN ASSESSMENT REPORT

UNIVERSITY SPEECH AND HEARING CLINIC **Boomtown, CA 90909**	**The name of the clinic, centered, all caps, bold Level 1 Heading (L1H)**
DIAGNOSTIC REPORT	**The type of report (L1H)**

CLIENT: Lynda Pen	**BIRTHDATE**: September 10, 1985	
ADDRESS: 555 N. Cedar #000	**CLINIC FILE NUMBER**: 87003	
CITY: Fresno, CA 93726	**DIAGNOSIS:** Language and Articulation Disorders	Identifying Information Arrange as shown.
TELEPHONE NUMBER: 555-0634	**DATE OF REPORT:** September 20, 1992	
REFERRED BY:	**CLINICIAN:**	

Report	Elements
BACKGROUND AND REASONS FOR REFERRAL	**L1H**
On September 15, 1993, Lynda Pen, a 7-year-old female, was referred to the University Speech and Hearing Clinic by Dr. James Osborne, a pediatrician. Lynda's delayed expressive speech was the reason for referral.	Indented (5 spaces) paragraphs Describe when, who, and how old a person was referred to which clinic and why.

Report	Elements
BACKGROUND AND REASONS FOR REFERRAL	**(L1H)**
HISTORY	**(L1H)**
Prrenatal and Birth History	**Flush Left Level 2 Heading, Bold (L2H)**
Mrs. Pen reported that she experienced preeclampsia five months into her pregnancy. At 30 weeks of gestation, Lynda was delivered by a Cesarean section. Birthweight was 5 pounds and 8 ounces. Because of numerous cardiac murmurs and a premature birth, Lynda did not thrive during her first six months of development.	Start with prenatal and birth history. Mother's health during pregnancy. Birth: normal or otherwise. Early development. Health during infancy and early childhood.
Developmental History	**(L2H)**
Lynda's developmental milestones were reported to be delayed for both physical and communicative behaviors. Mrs. Pen reported that Lynda walked at 26 months and "used a few single words" at 24 months. Mrs. Pen stated that currently, Lynda's speech consists of 10-15 word approximations.	Describe later development and physical growth. Communicative behaviors. Current status.

Report	Elements
Medical History	**(L2H)**
Mrs. Pen reported that Lynda had a single instance of otitis media at 9 months of age. At 10 months of age, Lynda underwent a specialized heart surgery called pulmonary banding to "prevent damage to her lungs." At 2 years of age, Lynda was operated on at the University of California Hospital in San Francisco by Drs. T. S. Musclemouster and O. S. Housterhouter for anterior skull reconstruction. At the age of 2 years and 2 months, Lynda underwent open heart surgery to repair numerous cardiac murmurs. The Medical Genetics Team at Valley Children's Hospital has reported that Lynda has a probable chromosome abnormality with extra material on chromosome 14q.	Summarize significant medical history, especially sensory problems. Medical and surgical treatment. Any previously made diagnostic statements.
Family, Social, and Educational History	**(L2H)**
Mrs. Pen does not recall any members of her family or those of her husband's family as having speech or language problems. Lynda is the only child of Mr. and Mrs. Pen. Mr. Pen is a high school teacher, and Mrs. Pen is an insurance underwriter. Lynda's grandmother, who lives with Mr. and Mrs. Pen, usually watches her when the parents are at work. Lynda sometimes plays with a younger child in the neighborhood. According to Mrs. Pen, Lynda plays cooperatively with children who are younger than she is.	Describe the family history of communicative problems. Describe the family. How many children? Patients' education and occupation. Who takes care of the child? Child's companions and play activities.

Report	Elements
Lynda attended the clinic of Exceptional Parents Unlimited from May, 1987 to April, 1988. Mrs. Pen reported that Lynda interacted well with her peers though the frequency of her social interactions were limited. Lynda is not currently attending school.	Describe the previous clinical and education program of relevance and the current educational level
ASSESSMENT INFORMATION	**(L1H)**
Orofacial Examination	**(L2H)**
An orofacial examination was conducted to evaluate the structural and functional integrity of the oral-facial mechanism. The examination revealed a broad nasal bridge and prominent epicanthal folds. Dental occlusion was marked by a Class III malocclusion. During smiling, there was bilateral retraction at the angle of the mouth. A narrow, inverted v-shaped palate was also noted. Due to Lynda's lack of cooperation, movements of the velum and the lateral pharyngeal walls were not observed. Labial and lingual mobility were deemed adequate for normal speech production.	Describe the orofacial examination: Integrity of oral and facial structures. Give a general description of the face, mouth, tongue, teeth, hard and soft palate, and movement of the soft palate and the tongue.
Speech Production and Intelligibility	**(L2H)**
Lynda's speech was assessed through a standardized test and a recorded conversational speech sample. To assess Lynda's speech production in fixed word positions, the Goldman-Fristoe Test of Articulation was administered. Her performance on the Goldman-Fristoe Test revealed numerous errors of articulation as summarized in the following table.	First say how speech production was assessed. Give the full name of tests administered. Do not ignore speech samples.

Report				Elements

	Initial	Medial	Final	
Substitutions	t/s; d/p	s/z		List errors of articulation noted on the test or tests administered.
	d/dr; k/kr; p/pl; s/sl; t/tr			
Omissions	/f, v, t, n, s, z, l, r, w, h, fl, st/	/b, m, f, d, n, s, l, r/	/p, b, m, f, v, t, n, s, r, k/	Arrange the errors of articulation in a table as shown.
Distortions	/s/			

A 90-utterance speech sample was tape recorded. An analysis of this sample revealed the following additional errors:

Describe the speech sample.

	Initial	Medial	Final	
Substitutions	p/b; b/m; t/s; y/l			List the errors of articulation noted in the speech sample.
Omissions	/m, k/	/g/	/d, l, k,/	Arrange the errors of articulation in a table like this.
	ts; fl		ts	
Distortions	/z, s/			

Report	Elements
Because of her numerous errors of articulation, Lynda's speech was generally unintelligible. With contextual cues present, her speech intelligibility was only 11.9% on a word-by-word and an utterance-by-utterance basis.	Describe the effects of articulation errors on intelligibility.
Language Production and Comprehension	**(L2H)**
Lynda's language production was assessed mainly through a language sample. She responded to questions and was asked to describe pictures in storybooks. Through this method, a 90-utterance language sample was obtained. An analysis of this sample showed a Mean Length of Utterance (MLU) of 1.13 for words. She did not produce any syntactically complete sentences as she said mostly one-word phrases. Because of reduced speech intelligibility marked by sound substitutions and omissions, Lynda's use of morphologic features could not be assessed.	Describe how you assessed language production. Give names of tests you administered. Describe the method of analysis.
	Describe the results of analysis. Describe limitations (something not done).
Lynda's comprehension of words was assessed by administering the Assessment of Children's Language Comprehension (ACLC). The following results were obtained: Part A: 76%; Part B: 80%; Part C: 10%; and Part D: 20%. These results suggest that her comprehension of words is poor.	Describe how you assessed comprehension. Describe the results.

Report	Elements
Voice and Fluency Based on the clinical observations, Lynda's vocal pitch and intensity were judged appropriate for her age. Because of her limited speech and language production, Lynda's fluency also was limited. However, clinically significant amounts or durations of dysfluencies were not observed.	**(L2H)** Comment on voice and fluency. Say your judgments were made on the basis of speech sample or samples.
DIAGNOSTIC SUMMARY The overall results of the assessment of Lynda Pen's speech and language production shows severe articulation and expressive language difficulties. Lynda's speech was characterized by reduced intelligibility due to many omitted and substituted phonemes and inconsistent production of others. Expressive language was limited mostly to one word utterances. This resulted in limited fluency though her vocal characteristics were within the limits of normal variations. Lynda's low scores on the ACLC suggest that her comprehension of language also was limited.	**(L1H)** Summarize the communicative problems noted in the assessment. Highlight the major problems that may be the targets for immediate intervention.

Report	Elements
RECOMMENDATIONS	**(L1H)**
It is recommended that Lynda Pen receive treatment for her speech and language problems. Among others to be determined later, the treatment targets may include the following:	Do you recommend treatment? What are some of the priority treatment targets?
1. Spontaneous naming of pictures of her family members with 90% accuracy. 2. Spontaneous naming of selected, functional words with 90% accuracy. 3. Production of phrases and sentences in a carefully graded sequence. 4. Correct production of selected phonemes.	List the potential targets as shown. List as many targets as seem appropriate.

Submitted by: _____
 	
      LaTeena LeBueque, B.A.
      Student Clinician
 	
Approved by: _____
      Benton Q. Bentley, M.A., CCC-SP
      Clinical Supervisor
	Name and signature of the student clinician
	
	Name and signature of the supervisor

Note to Student Clinicians

Because each clinic has its own format of writing clinical reports, student clinicians should study the format of their clinic. Examples given in this book are generic, with some commonly observed variations.

C.1.4. SAMPLE DIAGNOSTIC REPORTS

Note to Student Clinicians

On the following pages, you will see samples of diagnostic (assessment) reports. Study them for the general content and format of diagnostic reports. Compare the samples with the format used in your clinic.

C.1.4. SAMPLE DIAGNOSTIC REPORT: *ARTICULATION DISORDER*

UNIVERSITY SPEECH AND HEARING CLINIC
MIDSTATE UNIVERSITY
Middletown, Montana

DIAGNOSTIC REPORT

CLIENT: Pennifer Forbes

ADDRESS: 1326 E. Harvard

CITY: Middletown, Montana

TELEPHONE NUMBER: 555-0719

REFERRED BY: Dr. Pendelton

BIRTHDATE: January 14, 1987

CLINIC FILE NUMBER: 9-QR101

DATE OF REPORT: 2-06-92

DIAGNOSIS: Articulation/Phonological Disorder

CLINICIAN: Missouline Montoya

BACKGROUND AND REASONS FOR REFERRAL

Pennifer Forbes, a 5-year-old female, was seen on February 6, 1992 for an evaluation at the Speech and Hearing Clinic at the Mid State University, Middletown, Montana. Dr. Pendelton, a pediatrician, referred her to the clinic because of her articulation problems. Pennifer was accompanied to the clinic by her mother, Mrs. Forbes, who served as the informant.

HISTORY

Mrs. Forbes reported that Pennifer's speech is difficult to understand. She said that Pennifer leaves out sounds in her speech resulting in such words as "nake" for "snake." Pennifer also substitutes one sound for another. According to the mother, Pennifer says "tat" for "cat." Pennifer has previously received speech therapy at Big Sky Speech and Hearing Center for remediation of her articulation disorder.

Pennifer's birth and developmental history is not remarkable. She has enjoyed good health with no diseases of significance.

Family, Social, and Educational History

Pennifer is the second of three children. Mrs. Forbes did not report a family history of communiative disorders. Mrs. Forbes, a high school graduate, manages a restaurant. Mr. Forbes who did not finish his high school, is a maintenance man with the local school district.

Pennifer attends a kindergarten school and is doing well. However, other students and the teacher have complained about her unintelligible speech.

Oral-Peripheral Examination

An oral-peripheral examination was performed to assess the function and integrity of the oral mechanism. Pennifer's lips and hard palate appeared symmetrical at rest. She was able to perform the labial and lingual tasks asked by the clinician. The anterior and posterior faucial pillars were within normal limits. Vertical movement of the pharyngeal wall was observed upon the phonation of /a/.

Speech Production and Intelligibility

To assess Pennifer's speech sound production, a conversational speech sample was recorded. In addition, the Goldman Fristoe Test of Articulation was administered to assess speech sounds in fixed positions. An analysis of the speech sample and Pennifer's performance on the Goldman Fristoe Test revealed the following errors:

	Initial	Medial	Final
Substitutions	/s/ for /k/; /d/ for /g/ /t/ for /s/; /w/ for /r/ /b/ for /f/; /t/ for /ch/ /t/ for /sh/, /j/ for /z/ /b/ for /bl/, /b/ for /br/, /d/ for /dr/, /bl/ for /fl/, /t/ for /kl/, /l/ for /sl/, /d/ for /st/	/l/ for /t/; /t/ for /sh/ /b/ for /v/; /d/ for /g/; /b/ for /f/; /t/ for /ch/	/k/ for /t/
Omissions		/k/ /th/	/g/, /k/, /d/, /f/, /s/, /t/, /sh/, /ch/, /th/, /l/, /d/, /z/, /p/
Distortions		/z/	

The Khan-Lewis Phonological Analysis was administered to assess Pennifer's phonological error patterns. Pennifer's overall score of 32 on the test was calculated into an age equivalency of 2 to 9 years. The analysis revealed the following phonological processes:

Deletion of final consonants

Initial voicing

Palatal fronting

Velar fronting

Stridency deletion

Stopping of affricates and fricatives

Cluster simplification

Final devoicing

Liquid simplification

Due to numerous errors of articulation, only 23% of Pennifer's sentences were intelligible. Also, most of her misarticulations were not stimulable. Pennifer correctly imitated only /k/, /g/, /s/, and /f/. However, a diadochokinetic test showed essentially normal rates.

Language Production and Comprehension

Pennifer's conversational speech during the interview and assessment showed essentially normal language structure and use except for several missing grammatical morphemes. It is possible that missing grammatical morphemes are due to missing sounds. The mean length of utterance (MLU) of her speech sample was 5.4 morphemes, which is within normal limits for her age.

Voice and Fluency

Though difficult to understand, Pennifer's speech had normal rhythm. The rate of dysfluencies was within the normal range. Therefore, no further analysis of the dysfluency rate was made. Also, Pennifer's voice was judged normal.

DIAGNOSTIC SUMMARY

Pennifer Forbes exhibits a severe articulation disorder characterized by multiple misarticulations and limited speech intelligibility. Unless treated, her articulation disorder is likely to have negative social and educational consequences. Because Pennifer was stimulable for some of the consonants, the prognosis for improvement is judged to be good.

RECOMMENDATIONS

It is recommended that Pennifer receive treatment for her articulation disorder. As articulation and intelligibility improves, Pennifer's language may be further evaluated to see if morphological features emerge. If they do not, language treatment should be offered.

Submitted by: _____

             Missouline Montoya, B.A.

             Student Clinician

Approved by:_____

             Akbar Jamal, CCC-SP

             Speech-Language Pathologist

             Clinical Supervisor

C.1.4. SAMPLE DIAGNOSTIC REPORT: *VOICE DISORDER*

BALMTOWN UNIVERSITY SPEECH AND HEARING CLINIC

BALMTOWN, NEW YORK

DIAGNOSTIC REPORT

NAME: VALINE WRENN

BIRTHDATE: 9-10-59

AGE: 28

ADDRESS: 1919 S. Dakota #Q108-R

CITY: Fresno, CA 98705

TELEPHONE: 555-0608

DATE OF EXAMINATION: 2-9-88

CLINICAL CLASSIFICATION: VOICE DISORDER

CLINIC FILE NO: 08A-7314

REFERRED BY: DR. HANNA EISMER

EXAMINER: JANINA PRESHAM

INFORMANT: SELF

BACKGROUND AND PRESENTING COMPLAINTS

Valine Wrenn, a 28 year old female, was seen for a speech and language evaluation at the Balmtown University Speech and Hearing Clinic. She was referred to the clinic by her otolaryngologist, Dr. Eismer. Her presenting complaints were difficulty speaking loudly and difficulty speaking for long periods of time. She also noted a "lack of excitement" in her voice and difficulty producing sounds at the ends of sentences due to a low pitch. Valine came to the Clinic by herself and provided all the information.

HISTORY

Early History

Valine reported that her voice had sounded "funny" since early childhood. During her high school years, she became aware of a low pitch and monotone quality after listening to herself on audio tape. Valine did not recall previous consultations or treatment for her voice problem. According to Valine, her developmental history was unremarkable.

Medical History

On November 3, 1987, Valine received a medical evaluation by Dr. Hanna Eismer, an otolaryngologist. Dr. Eismer reported Valine as having normal external auditory canals and tympanic membranes. The nose and oral cavities were also clear. A fiberoptic endoscope was used to examine Valine's larynx. Vocal fold structure and motion were reported to be normal. There was no evidence of vocal nodules or lesions. The vocal folds were described as being very minimally erythematous and slightly swollen on the free edge.

Valine reported having allergies to molds, trees, and grasses. These allergies affected her only when she was in close proximity to one of the allergens, causing excessive phlegm in the throat and postnasal drip. Valine recently began using Beconase (an inhalant) to relieve the allergies. Valine also had excessive colds resulting in phlegm and postnasal drip. These were noted as occurring approximately once a month beginning in October or November, and lasting about a week. Valine expressed the opinion that the colds were caused by stress and emotional problems. She temporarily discontinued the use of the Beconase while using Afrin and Neo-Synephrine for the colds. Excessive phlegm resulted in frequent coughing and throat clearing. Recently, Valine has made an attempt to decrease these vocally abusive behaviors.

Family, Social, and Educational History

Valine is a student at the Balmtown University, Balmtown, New York, majoring in speech communication. She is divorced and lives with her 3-year-old daughter, Haline. Either the television or the radio is on in Valine's apartment for the majority of the time she is at home. While speaking to her daughter, Valine rarely shouts through the apartment. Instead, she makes an effort to go in to the room where her daughter is. Valine noted that she frequently sings for personal pleasure. She sings in numerous and varied settings, including at home, in the car, and on campus. She reported that she rarely yells. She has between 2-5 telephone conversations per day, ranging from 2 to 30 minutes in length. Valine stated that she does not habitually drink coffee, tea, soft drinks, or alcoholic beverages. She does drink at least two glasses of low–fat milk every day. Valine mentioned that friends easily identify her voice and describe it as being "low and sexy."

Valine typically experiences a feeling of tightness in the throat when nervous, as well as a higher pitch, lower intensity, and difficulty projecting her voice.

ASSESSMENT INFORMATION

Orofacial Examination

An orofacial examination was conducted to assess the integrity of oral and facial structures. Valine's facial features appeared symmetrical, with lingual and labial mobility adequate for speech. However, restricted oral mobility was noted during speech. Velopharyngeal closure was acoustically deemed adequate during repeated productions of /a/. Diadochokinetic rates were within normal limits.

Hearing Screening

Using a Maico portable screening audiometer (model MA-20A), Valine's hearing was screened at 25 dB for 250, 500, 1000, 2000, 4000, and 8000 Hz. At all frequencies, Valine passed the screening bilaterally.

Speech Production and Comprehension

Valine's speech production and comprehension were informally assessed. Her conversational speech and her interaction during the interview did not reveal speech production or comprehension problems. Therefore, these aspects of her communicative behaviors were judged to be within normal variations.

Language and Fluency

Valine's language and fluency were assessed informally. Her conversational speech during the assessment period did not suggest problems of language structure or use. Her fluency and rates of dysfluencies also were judged to be within normal variations.

Voice

Valine's fundamental frequency ranged between 150 Hz and 200 Hz on the fundamental frequency indicator. This pitch was determined to be low for Valine's gender and stature. During the interview, frequent glottal fry and hoarseness of voice were observed. A later analysis of the audiotaped speech sample revealed that glottal fry and hoarseness were more likely to occur on downward inflections of most utterances. On approximately 60% of her utterances, either glottal fry, hoarseness, or both were observed. However, Valine's breath support appeared adequate for speech.

DIAGNOSTIC SUMMARY

Valine Wrenn's history suggests vocally abusive behaviors. She used a habitual pitch that is too low for her. This may have resulted in excessive glottal fry. She also used a low vocal focus which may have adversely affected the extent to which she could project her voice.

RECOMMENDATIONS

It was recommended that Valine Wrenn receive voice therapy. Specific recommendations include:

1. Eliminating glottal fry by raising the client's habitual pitch to a more optimal pitch during spontaneous conversational speech produced in nonclinical settings.

2. Decreasing such abusive vocal behaviors as ineffective management of colds and allergies, improper fluid intake, and singing and speaking in noisy situations.

Submitted by: _____
                    Janina Presham, B.A.
                    Student Clinician

Approved by: _____
                    Dambly Doumbleson, M.A., CCC-SP
                    Clinical Supervisor and Speech-Language Pathologist

---

C.1.4. SAMPLE DIAGNOSTIC REPORT: *APHASIA AND APRAXIA*

UNIVERSITY SPEECH AND HEARING CLINIC

Tinkyville, Tennessee

DIAGNOSTIC REPORT

NAME: Lynn M. Zoolanfoos

BIRTHDATE: 12-27-46

ADDRESS: 111 E. Cornell

CLINIC FILE NUMBER: 910019

CITY: Tinkyville, TN 43704

DIAGNOSIS: Aphasia and Apraxia

TELEPHONE NUMBER: 229-9850

DATE OF REPORT: 9-27-92

CLINICIAN: Maxine Traoumer

SUPERVISOR: Galaxy Galvestrouton, M.A., CCC-SP

REFERRED BY: Dr. Mendelsohn

ASSESSMENT DATE: 9-24-92

BACKGROUND AND REASONS FOR REFERRAL

Lynn Zoolanfoos, a 44-year-old female, was referred to the Speech and Hearing Clinic at the Tinkyville State University in Tinkyville, Tennessee. Her physician, Dr. Muskwhiter Mendelsohn referred her for a speech-language evaluation following a stroke.

Lynn's speech and language were evaluated in two sessions. She was seen on September 27, 1991 and October 10, 1991. Lynn was unaccompanied to the diagnostic sessions. Lynn suffered an initial stroke in July of 1990. On September 30, 1990, she experienced a second stroke which resulted in right hemiplegia, expressive and receptive aphasia, and verbal apraxia.

HISTORY

Medical History

Lynn was diagnosed with atopic dermatitis at 3 months of age which is characterized by itchy, red elevated areas on the skin and scratching.   Lynn has a history of heart problems. She resides with her mother, Gladys Miller, who experiences severe emphysema and is on continuous oxygen. Lynn and her mother have a home care aide who comes into the home 6 hours daily.

Lynn reported she wears braces on her right leg and right hand and uses a cane to assist with walking.   Lynn enjoys activities such as bowling and watching television. She now wants to improve her writing skills.

Previous Speech and Language Services

For the past 6 months, Lynn has received speech and language services at the Community Hospital Speech and Hearing Department. Previous treatment targets include the production of two- to four- word phrases; correct production of initial and final consonants in single words; auditory comprehension of two- and three-step directions and two- and three-element questions; and reading comprehension of three- to six- word sentences.

ASSESSMENT INFORMATION

Lynn cooperated during the evaluation and showed excellent motivation for continuing therapy. She showed a keen interest in the assessment tasks presented to her. She said that she wanted to improve her speech and language skills.

Orofacial Examination

An orofacial examination was performed to evaluate the functional and structural integrity of the oral-facial complex. Facial features including lips at rest were judged to be symmetrical and normal in appearance and function. The tongue was normal in appearance, but its lateral movements were sluggish. There were groping behaviors while attempting to draw the tip of the tongue along the hard palate. A slight neutroclusion was noted. The hard palate was narrow, with a high arch and a small bony outgrowth along the midline. Pronounced rugae was evident in the premaxillary region. The soft palate was of adequate length and elevated vertically and posteriorly to achieve closure. Velopharyngeal functioning was acoustically judged to be adequate during production of /a/. An assessment of diadochokinetic rates revealed slowness suggesting weakness in circumoral and lingual musculature. The productions also were characterized by substitutions suggesting verbal apraxia.

Voice

Lynn's voice characteristics were subjectively judged based on her conversational speech. Except for a hyponasal resonance, her voice was judged normal.

Hearing Screening

A hearing screening was performed bilaterally at 25 dB HL for 250, 500, 1000, 2000, 4000, and 8000 Hz. Lynn passed at all frequencies bilaterally.

Speech Production

The Apraxia Battery for Adults was administered to verify the presence of apraxia and provide a rough estimate of the severity of the disorder. The summary of scores were as follows:

Subtest I	Diadochokinetic Rate
p t	13
t k	10
p t k	6
Subtest II	Increasing Word Length
1 syllable average	1.8
2 syllable average	1.7
3 syllable average	1.9
Deterioration in performance score	0
Subtest III	Limb Apraxia and Oral Apraxia
Limb Apraxia	34
Oral Apraxia	39
Subtest IV	Latency and Utterance Time for Polysyllabic Words
Latency Time	93 seconds
Utterance Time	2 seconds
	Repeated Trials Test
Subtest V	
Total Amount of Change	+1
Subtest VI	Inventory of Articulation Characteristics of Apraxia
Total YES Items	2

Evaluation of Lynn's performance on the subtests reveals searching behaviors for making gestures and a low score on articulation characteristics of apraxia.

Language Production and Comprehension

A 76-utterance, 157-word language sample was obtained. The Mean-Length-of-Utterance for these utterances was 2.19 for words and 2.42 for morphemes. Word finding difficulties were noted. Automatic speech was evident in some of her replies.

To make an initial assessment of Lynn's aphasia, the first three items of each subtest of the Western Aphasia Battery were administered as a screening test. In the following table, Lynn's scores are listed in the left-hand column. Several subtests were scored beyond the first three items. These scores are listed in the right-hand column. The scores were as follows:

	Client's Subscores on first three items/ Maximum	Client's Subscores beyond first three items/ Maximum
Spontaneous Speech		
Information Content	6/10	
Fluency	5/10	
Yes/No Questions	9/9	36/42
Auditory Word Recognition	9/27	
Sequential Commands	6/6	8/22
Repetition	6/6	60/70
Word Fluency	2/20	
Sentence Completion	4/6	6/10
Responsive Speech	0/6	
Reading	20.5/32	30.5/52
Writing	31.5/100	
Praxis	6/6	27/30
Drawing	3/9	
Calculation	0/4	

Lynn performed well on tasks involving auditory comprehension for Yes/No questions, auditory comprehension of one-part sequential commands, verbal repetition of single words and two- to five- word phrases, sentence completion, and reading single words. Errors were noted during tasks involving oral reading of phrases and sentences, spelling, writing (except for writing numbers and her own name and copying printed words), calculation, drawing, responsive speech, word fluency, auditory word recognition, spontaneous speech, and two-part sequential commands. Lynn's performance on the Praxis subtest did not suggest oral or verbal apraxia. An Aphasia Quotient and a Cortical Quotient were unobtainable due to partial presentation of the test.

DIAGNOSTIC SUMMARY

Lynn's performance on various assessment tasks suggests a moderate to severe expressive and receptive aphasia with anomia. A mild verbal apraxia is also suggested.

RECOMMENDATIONS

Speech and language treatment is recommended for Lynn. Immediate treatment goals recommended for Lynn include the following:

1. Improve expressive language.
2. Teach consistent productions of selected functional words and phrases. These productions may include a variety of communication modes (gesturing, drawing, speaking, writing) to improve communicative effectiveness.
3. Teach four- to six- word sentence completion performance with 90% accuracy.
4. Improve receptive language in reading
5. Teach correct responses to questions about silently read material with 90% accuracy.

Submitted by_____
        Maxine Traoumer, B.A.
        Student Clinician

Approved by_____
        Galaxy Galvestrouton, M.A., CCC-SP
        Clinical Supervisor

C.1.4. SAMPLE DIAGNOSTIC REPORT: *STUTTERING*

UNIVERSITY SPEECH AND HEARING CLINIC
FREEMONT UNIVERSITY
Valleyville, California

DIAGNOSTIC REPORT

NAME: James Foxx   ASSESSMENT DATE: February 2, 1992

BIRTHDATE: January 26, 1971   FILE NUMBER: RS92019

ADDRESS: Graves 312 B   DIAGNOSIS: Stuttering

CITY: Valleyville, CA 90710-3342   DATE OF REPORT: February 5, 1992

TELEPHONE NUMBER: 555-3235   INFORMANT: Self

REFERRED BY: SELF   CLINICIAN: Meena Wong

BACKGROUND AND PRESENTING COMPLAINT

James Foxx, a 21-year-old male, was seen for a speech and language evaluation at the Freemont University Speech and Hearing Clinic on February 5, 1992. He had applied for services after he read an article in the campus newspaper about the speech and hearing services on campus. The reason for seeking services was his stuttering. James is a student at the university, majoring in computer science.

HISTORY

James reported that according to what his parents have told him, his stuttering began when he was about 3 years of age.   From the age of 4 through 9 years, James received treatment for his stuttering at J.R. Cronin Elementary School in Dublin, California. At age 7, he also received approximately a year of treatment at California State University, Stanislaus. He has not received treatment since that time. James reported that the severity of his stuttering fluctuates depending on his mood, and it is more pronounced in stressful situations.

He reports increased frequency of stuttering when he speaks to strangers, his instructors, and his father. He thinks he is less dysfluent when he speaks to his mother, brother, sister, and close friends. He said that he would rather not order at restaurants, buy tickets at counters, introduce himself, or answer telephone calls. He does not think that he has difficulty with specific words or sounds.

Family and Social History

James lives on campus. His parents live in Merced, California. He comes from a family of three children. He is the oldest. His younger brother and younger sister do not have communication problems. He believes that his maternal uncle and his son both stutter. James is not aware of any person on his father's side who stutters.

James lives with a roommate in a dorm on the campus. He says that his verbal interactions with his roommate are limited. He has other friends with whom he spends more time. Reportedly, he has difficulty asking for dates because he is worried that he might stutter badly.

Educational and Occupational History

James had part-time jobs in various businesses. He believes that his stuttering was always a frustrating problem in the work place. He usually avoided speaking to his supervisors. He tended to seek work that did not involve too much oral communication.

James is studying for a degree in computer science. He is doing well in his courses. He does not think that his stuttering has negatively affected his coursework or relationship with his instructors. He plans to work for a private company when he finished his degree. He is concerned about being able to communicate under job pressure. James appears to be highly motivated for treatment as he wants to be able to speak fluently.

ASSESSMENT INFORMATION

Orofacial Examination

An orofacial examination was performed to assess the structural and functional integrity of the oral mechanism. The examination did not reveal anything of clinical significance.

Types and Frequency of Dysfluencies

To analyze the types and the frequency of dysfluencies, a conversational speech sample was recorded. James was also asked to bring an audiotaped conversational speech sample within he next 3 days. An analysis of the two samples revealed the following types and frequency of dysfluencies.

	Clinic Sample Total Words: 1231		Home Sample Total Words: 1071	
Dysfluency Types	Frequency of Dysfluency	% of Total Dysfluency	Frequency of Dysfluency	% of Total Dysfluency
Interjections	86	6.9	26	2.4
Pauses	29	2.3	9	0.8
Part-word reps	68	5.5	60	5.6
Whole-word reps	9	7	57	5.3
Audible prolongations	52	4.2	4	0.4
Silent prolongations	7	0.6	4	0.4
Revisions	8	6	6	0.6
Incomplete phrases	2	0.2	1	0.1
TOTAL	**261**		**199**	
PERCENT DYS. RATE	**21**		**18.6**	

Both the speech samples contained pauses from 5–25 seconds in duration. His sound and silent prolongations typically exceeded 1 sec. James' rate of speech was calculated between 110 and 150 words per minute depending on the amount and duration of pauses and prolongations. He intermittently rushed groups of words. Overall rate of speech was variable depending on amount of dysfluencies.

An occasional eye blink and hand movements were observed during the interview. These motor behaviors were most often associated with part-word repetitions and silent and sound prolongations.

Language Production and Comprehension

An informal assessment of a 100-utterance, 1,231-word, conversational language sample revealed expressive language skills that were judged appropriate for his level of education. No language comprehension problems were noted during the interview.

Voice

James spoke with laryngeal tension and hard glottal attack approximately 50% of the time. However, he exhibited appropriate vocal intensity, intonation, and inflectional patterns.

Hearing Screening

A bilateral hearing screening was administered at 25 dB HL for 250, 500, 1000, 2000, 4000, 6000, and 8000 Hz. James responded to all frequencies.

DIAGNOSTIC SUMMARY

Analysis of the conversational speech samples revealed that James Foxx exhibits a severe fluency disorder. His dominant dysfluencies are repetitions, prolongations, interjections, and pauses.

RECOMMENDATIONS

It is recommended that James Foxx receive treatment for his stuttering. The Fluency-Chain Reinforcement Technique may be used. Treatment should focus on the following:

1.   Teaching appropriate airflow, rate reduction, and gentle phonatory onset.

2.   Production of 98% fluent speech within the clinic.

3.   Maintenance of at least 95% fluency in extraclinical situations.

Submitted by:_____
                    Meena Wong, B.A.
                    Student Clinician

Approved by:_____
                    Nancy Lopez, M.A., CCC-SP
                    Clinical Supervisor

Note to Student Clinicians

In practicing diagnostic report writing in the next section, use the information given on the left-hand pages and write your report on the right-hand pages. Give appropriate headings and subheadings. Invent missing information.

C.1.5. PRACTICE IN CLINICAL REPORT WRITING

C.1.5. ASSESSMENT REPORT: *ARTICULATION DISORDER*

Data Sheet

Name of the clinic, city, and state: (invent)	Write the name and address of the clinic **(L1H)**
DIAGNOSTIC REPORT Mathew Moon, client; age, 8; address: (invent) telephone: (invent); Jenny Soon, clinician; date of assessment: (invent); diagnosis: Articulation Disorder; referred by Dr. Lydia Bong, a counselor.	What kind of report? **(L1H)** Identifying information Arrange appropriately
BACKGROUND AND REASONS FOR REFERRAL Use the information above No prior assessment Informant: father	**(L1H)** Who, how old a person, referred when, to which clinic, and why?

Write your report. Invent information as needed

Write the name and
address of the clinic
(L1H)

What kind of report?

(L1H)

Identifying information

Arrange appropriately

**Write the L1H that
goes here.**

Indented paragraphs.

When, who, and how
old a person was
referred to which clinic,
and why?

Data Sheet

HISTORY	**(L1H)**
Birth and Development	**(L2H)**
Normal pregnancy, Cesarean delivery	Prenatal, birth
No other prenatal or natal complications	Mother's health
Normal infancy	Early development
Delayed motor development, but no specific information	
First words at 18 months	Early language
Soon language development somewhat accelerated to approximate the normal	development
Medical History	**(L2H)**
Frequent middle ear infections	Diseases of
Mild conductive loss according to previous clinical reports	significance
Frequent attacks of cold and allergies	
Chicken pox at 4	

Write your report. Invent information as needed

(L1H)

(L2H)

Prenatal, birth

Mother's health

Early development

Early language

development

(L2H)

Medical history

Diseases of

significance

Data Sheet

Family, Social, and Educational History   **(L2H)**

An older brother (10 years), a younger sister (2 years)

Family
How many children?

None with a communicative disorder

Any family history of
communicative
problems?

Mother: college graduate; a real estate broker
Father: high school graduate; car repairman

Parents' education and
occupation

Mathew, in 2nd grade, doing below average school work,
Was held back the first year in school

Educational
information

He plays well other children
Parents say he is cooperative, affectionate, well behaved
Gets group speech treatment at his school

Child's companions
and social behavior

Any other information
about the family

Write your report. Invent information as needed

(L2H)

Family
How many children?

Any family history of communicative problems?

Parents' education and occupation

Child's companions and social behavior

Any other information about the family

Data Sheet

ASSESSMENT INFORMATION	(L1H)

Orofacial Examination

(L2H)

Class II malocclusion

Sluggish lingual movements

No other findings of significance

Describe the orofacial examination: integrity of oral and facial structures.

Give a general description of the face, mouth, teeth, tongue, hard and soft palate, and movement of the soft palate and the tongue.

(L2H)

Hearing Screening

Screened: 250, 500, 1000, 2000, 4000, and 8000 Hz at 25 dBHL

Failed at all tested frequencies

Needs a complete audiological examination

What frequencies were screened and at what level?

What were the results?

Write your report. Invent information as needed

(L1H)

(L2H)

Describe the orofacial examination: integrity of oral and facial structures.

Give a general description of the face, mouth, teeth, tongue, hard and soft palate, and movement of the soft palate and the tongue.
(L2H)

What frequencies were screened and at what level?

What were the results?

Data Sheet

Speech Production and Intelligibility

Conversational speech

Goldman-Fristoe Test of Articulation

Numerous errors in both

In the initial position of words, omitted: /b, d, p, f, v, r, k/; substituted:

t/k; distorted: /z, s/

In the medial position of words, omitted: /b, m, f, z, s, l, g, r/

In the final position of words, omitted: /b, d, p, f, v, r, k, t, l, m, n, s/

The same errors in conversational speech

Intelligibility with contextual cues: 75% for utterances

(L2H)

How was speech
production assessed?

Give the full name of
tests administered.
Do not ignore speech
samples.

Summarize the errors
in a table.

What was the speech

intelligibility?

Write your report. Invent information as needed.

(L2H)
How was speech production assessed?

Give the full name of tests administered. Do not ignore speech samples.

Summarize the errors in a table.

What was the speech intelligibility?

Data Sheet

Language Production and Comprehension	**(L2H)**
Conversational speech sample: 120 utterances	How did you assess
Tests administered: Peabody Picture Vocabulary Test:	language production?
result indicating age-appropriate responses	
The Test for Auditory Comprehension of Language (TACL)	What tests?
Language comprehension: Age appropriate	
MLU: 3.0 words	
Analysis of conversational speech for missing grammatic features	How did you analyze
	the results?
Many morphologic features missing, but consider the errors of articulation	What were the results
(invent missing morphologic features)	of the analysis?
Limited sentence structures	
Voice and Fluency	**(L2H)**
	How did you assess
Informally assessed through conversational speech samples	voice and fluency?
Judged to be within normal limits	What is your
	evaluation?

Write your report. Invent information as needed

(L2H)

How did you assess language production?

What tests?

How did you analyze the results?

What were the results of the analysis?

(L2H)

How did you assess voice and fluency?

What is your evaluation?

Data Sheet

<table>
<tr><td>

DIAGNOSTIC SUMMARY

Multiple misarticulations

Speech intelligibility: 75%

Normal voice and fluency

Limited language structures; many missing morphologic features

RECOMMENDATIONS

Treatment recommended

Goal is to teach the misarticulated phonemes

A later, more detailed language assessment

Parent training in maintenance

Submitted by_____ (Your name)

Approved by _____ (Clinical supervisor)

</td><td>

(L1H)

Summarize the communicative problems.

(L1H)

Do you recommend treatment?

What are the priority treatment targets?

Who submitted the report?

Write the name, degree, and title.

Who approved the report?

Write the name, degree, certification, and title.

</td></tr>
</table>

Write your report. Invent information as needed

(L1H)

Summarize the communicative problems.

(L1H)

Do you recommend treatment?
What are the priority treatment targets?

Who submitted the report?
Write the name, degree, and title.

Who approved the report?
Write the name, degree, certification, and title.

C.1.5. ASSESSMENT REPORT: *LANGUAGE DISORDERS*

Data Sheet

Name of the clinic, city, and state: (invent)

(L1H)

Write the name and address of the clinic.

DIAGNOSTIC REPORT

(L1H)

What kind of report?

Sylvia Sun, client; age, 5; address:

(invent) telephone: (invent); Jenny Soon, clinician; date of assessment:

(invent); diagnosis: Language Disorder; referred by Dr. Chang

Loongson, a physician.

Identifying information
Arrange appropriately

BACKGROUND AND REASONS FOR REFERRAL

(L1H)

Use the information above
No prior assessment
Informant: mother

Who, how old a person, referred when, to which clinic and why?

Write your report. Invent information as needed

(L1H)
Write the name and address of the clinic.

What kind of report?

(L2H)

Identifying information

Arrange appropriately

Write the L1H that goes here.

Indented paragraphs

When, who, and how old a person was referred to which clinic and why?

Data Sheet

HISTORY	**(L1H)**
Birth and Development	**(L2H)**
Normal pregnancy, delivery	Prenatal, birth
No significant prenatal or natal complications	Mother's health
Normal infancy	Early development
Delayed language, motor development	Early language
First words at 22 months	development
Two-word phrases not until 28 months	
Errors of articulation	
"Does not speak in complete sentences" (mother)	
"Does not know many words" (mother)	
Medical History	**(L2H)**
One episode of high fever and convulsions at age 16 months	Diseases of
Prone to frequent episodes of cough, cold, and allergic reactions	significance
Chicken pox at 4	
Slow physical growth	

Write your report. Invent information as needed.

(L1H)

(L2H)

Prenatal, birth

Mother's health

Early development

Early language

development

(L2H)

Medical history

Diseases of

significance

Data Sheet

Family, Social, and Educational History	**(L2H)**
An older sister (8 years), a younger brother (3 years) Sister is diagnosed as mentally retarded, enrolled in special education No parental concern about the younger brother's speech and language	**Family** How many children?
Older sister is language delayed, getting treated in school	Any family history of communicative problems?
Mother: a high school graduate; a receptionist in an auto body repair shop Father: high school graduate; plumber	Parent's education and occupation
Enrolled in a kindergarten program Needs special attention	Educational information
Does not play cooperatively A few companions who are much younger	Child's companions and social behavior Any other information about the family

Write your report. Invent information as needed.

(L2H)
Family How many children?
Any family history of communicative problems?
Parents' education and occupation
Educational information
Child's companions and social behavior
Any other information about the family

Data Sheet

ASSESSMENT INFORMATION	**(L1H)**
Orofacial Examination	**(L2H)**
No malocclusion Sluggish lingual movements Slow diadochokinetic rate No other findings of significance	Describe the orofacial examination: integrity of oral and facial structures. Give a general description of the face, mouth, teeth, tongue, hard and soft palate, and movement of the soft palate and the tongue.
Hearing Screening	**(L2H)**
Screened: 250, 500, 1000, 2000, 4000, and 8000 Hz at 25 dBHL Passed at all tested frequencies	What frequencies were screened and at what level? What were the results?

Write your report. Invent information as needed

(L1H)

(L2H)

Describe the orofacial examination: integrity of oral and facial structures

Give a general description of the face, mouth, teeth, tongue, hard and soft palate, and movement of the soft palate and the tongue.

(L2H)

What frequencies were screened and at what level?

What were the results?

Data Sheet

Speech Production and Intelligibility	**(L2H)**
	How was speech production assessed?
Conversational speech	
Templin-Darley Test of Articulation	Give the full name of tests administered. Do not ignore speech samples.
Numerous errors in both	
In the initial position of words, omitted: /b, d, t, l, g, m, n, k/; distorted: /z, s/	Summarize the errors in a table.
In the medial position of words, omitted: /b, m, f, z, s, l, g, r/	
In the final position of words, omitted: /b, d, p, r, k, t, m, n, s/	
The same errors in conversational speech	
Intelligibility with contextual cues: 80% for utterances	What was the speech intelligibility?

Write your report. Invent information as needed

(L2H)
How was speech production assessed?

Give the full name of tests administered. Do not ignore speech samples.

Summarize the errors in a table.

What was the speech intelligibility?

Data Sheet

Language Production and Comprehension

(L2H)

Conversational speech sample: 60 utterances

Shown pictures, objects, and toys to evoke language

The Assessment of Children's Language Comprehension (ACLC)

Language comprehension: Approximately that of a 3 year old

MLU: 4.0 words

How did you assess language production? What tests?

Analysis of conversational speech for missing grammatic features and pragmatic functions

How did you analyze the results?

Limited vocabulary

Many morphologic features missing

(invent missing morphologic features)

Typically, three- to four-word utterances

Few grammatically complete sentences

Limited sentence structures

Difficulty in maintaining topic and conversational turn taking

What were the results of the analysis?

Voice and Fluency

(L2H)

Informally assessed through conversational speech samples

Limited fluency because of limited language

Voice judged to be within normal limits

How did you assess voice and fluency? What is your evaluation?

Write your report. Invent information as needed.

(L2H)

How did you assess language production?

What tests?

How did you analyze the results?

What were the results of the analysis?

(L2H)

How did you assess voice and fluency?

What is your evaluation?

Data Sheet

DIAGNOSTIC SUMMARY

Multiple misarticulations

Speech intelligibility: 80%

Normal voice but limited fluency

Limited vocabulary and language structures; many missing morphologic

features; pragmatic problems; deficiency in language comprehension

RECOMMENDATIONS

Treatment recommended

Initial goal is to expand vocabulary, teach early morphemes, and basic

sentence structures

Later goal is to teach correct articulation of phonemes, pragmatic features

A more detailed language assessment before initiating treatment

Parent training in a home treatment and maintenance program

Submitted by_____ (Your name)

Approved by _____ (Clinical supervisor)

(L1H)

Summarize the

communicative

problems.

(L1H)

Do you recommend

treatment?

What are the priority

treatment targets?

Who submitted the

report?

Write the name,

degree, and title.

Who approved the

report?

Write the name,

degree, certification,

and title.

Write your report. Invent information as needed

(L1H)

Summarize the communicative problems.

(L1H)

Do you recommend treatment?
What are the priority treatment targets?

Who submitted the report?
Write the name, degree, and title.

Who approved the report?
Write the name, degree, certification, and title.

C.1.5. ASSESSMENT REPORT: *STUTTERING*

Data Sheet

Name of the clinic, city, and state: (invent)

(L1H)
Write the name and
address of the clinic.

DIAGNOSTIC REPORT

Marvin Lenson, client; age, 32; address:
(invent) telephone: (invent); Barbara Bandit, clinician; date of
assessment: (invent); diagnosis: Stuttering; referral: Self

(L1H)
What kind of report?
Identifying information
Arrange appropriately

BACKGROUND AND REASONS FOR REFERRAL

Use the information above
Several prior assessments and treatments at various clinics with no
lasting effects
Informant: Self
Client reported that: stuttering started when he was about 5
Has had prior treatment throughout the school years
Does not recall treatment techniques
Stuttering varies across situations; but more stuttering when talking to
strangers; his boss; more fluent talking to wife; avoids telephones,
ordering in restaurants, and talking to groups

(L1H)

Who, how old a person,
referred when, to which
clinic and why?
Summarize the history
of stuttering.

Write your report. Invent information as needed.

(L1H)
Write the name and address of the clinic

(L1H)
What kind of report?

Identifying information.

Arrange appropriately

Write the L1H that goes here.

Indent paragraphs

When, who, and how old a person was referred to which clinic and why?

Summarize the history of stuttering.

Data Sheet

HISTORY	(L1H)
Birth and Development	(L2H)
Mother had told the client that everything was normal	Prenatal, birth
Reportedly normal	Mother's health
Normal infancy	Early development
Normal motor development	
Advanced early language development as told by parents	Early language
Considers himself verbally competent; likes to read and write; has good vocabulary and command of the language	development
Medical History	(L2H)
Nothing of clinical significance	Diseases of significance

Write your report. Invent information as needed.

(L1H)

(L2H)

Prenatal, birth
Mother's health
Early development

Early language
development

(L2H)

Medical history

Diseases of
significance

Data Sheet

Family, Social, and Educational History	**(L2H)**
An older brother (37 years), a younger sister (27 years), a younger brother (24 years),	Family How many children?
Older brother use to stutter, but has been mostly fluent for the past 10 years A maternal uncle (65) still stutters A paternal aunt (62) used to stutter, but has been fluent for many years No history of other communicative disorders	Any family history of communicative problems?
Both hold doctoral degrees Mother: a pediatrician Father: clinical psychologist	Parents' education and occupation
Client holds a master's degree in structural engineering Works for a construction company	Educational and occupational information
Married, wife owns a clothing store one daughter (3), speaks normally	Personal information

Write your report. Invent information as needed.

(L2H)
Family How many children?
Any family history of communicative problems?
Parents' education and occupation
Parents' education and occupation
Educational and occupational information
Personal information

Data Sheet

ASSESSMENT INFORMATION	**(L1H)**
Orofacial Examination Nothing of clinical significance	**(L2H)** Describe the orofacial examination: integrity of oral and facial structures.
Hearing Screening Screened: 250, 500, 1000, 2000, 4000, and 8000 Hz at 25 dBHL Passed the screening	**(L2H)** What frequencies were screened and at what level? What were the results?

Write your report. Invent information as needed.

(L1H)

(L2H)

Describe the orofacial
examination:
integrity of oral and
facial structures.
State the results.

(L2H)

What frequencies were
screened and at what
level?

What were the results?

Data Sheet

Speech and Language Production

Informally assessed as the client was interviewed

Judged to have normal articulation and superior language skills

Speech intelligibility 100% for utterances

Voice

Informally assessed as the client was interviewed

Vocal qualities judged to be normal

(L2H)

How were speech and language production assessed?

What was the speech intelligibility?

Summarize the observations.

(L2H)

How assessed?
Summarize the observations.

Write your report. Invent information as needed.

(L2H)
How were speech and language production assessed?

What was the speech intelligibility?

Summarize the observations.

(L2H)
How was voice assessed?
Summarize the observations.

Data Sheet

Assessment of Fluency

Conversational speech sample: 2,000 words

Oral reading sample: 500 words

Two home samples of at least 1,000 words each requested for later analysis

Analysis of types and frequency of dysfluencies (all types)

Calculation of percent dysfluency rate

Conversational speech:

Part-word reps: 57; sound prolongations: 48; syllable interjections: 28; whole-word reps: 39; pauses (1 sec or more): 45; broken words: 21

Total number of dysfluencies: 238

Percent dysfluency rate: 11.9

Oral reading:

Part-word reps: 42; sound prolongations: 39; syllable interjections: 34; whole-word reps: 53; pauses (1 sec or more): 54; broken words: 21

Total number of dysfluencies: 243

Percent dysfluency rate: 48.6

Eye blinks

knitting of the eyebrows

L2H

How did you assess fluency and stuttering?

How did you analyze the results?

What were the results of the analysis?

Describe the associated motor behaviors.

Write your report. Invent information as needed.

(L2H)

How did you assess fluency and stuttering?

How did you analyze the results?

What were the results of the analysis?

Describe associated motor behaviors

Data Sheet

DIAGNOSTIC SUMMARY

Clinically significant dysfluency rate: 11.9%

Part-word reps, sound prolongations, syllable interjections, whole-word reps, pauses, and broken words

Higher dysfluency rate in oral reading: 48.6

Few associated motor behaviors

(L1H)
Summarize the dysfluency rates. Specify the types.

RECOMMENDATIONS

Treatment recommended

Goal is to teach the skills of fluency (gentle phonatory onset, rate reduction through syllable prolongation, and appropriate airflow management)

Self-monitoring skills for maintenance

Submitted by_____ (Your name)

Approved by _____ (Clinical supervisor)

(L1H)
Do you recommend treatment?
What are the priority treatment targets?

Who submitted the report?
Write the name, degree, and title.
Who approved the report?
Write the name, degree, certification, and title.

Write your report. Invent information as needed.

(L1H)

Summarize the
dysfluency rates.
Specify the types.

(L1H)

Do you recommend
treatment?
What are the priority
treatment targets?

Who submitted the
report?
Write the name,
degree, and title.

Who approved the
report?
Write the name,
degree, certification,
and title.

C.1.5. ASSESSMENT REPORT: *VOICE DISORDER*

Data Sheet

Name of the clinic, city, and state: (invent)

(L1H)

Write the name and address of the clinic.

DIAGNOSTIC REPORT

(L1H)

What kind of report?

Raj Mohan, 35 years; address: (invent) telephone: (invent); clinician: yourself; date of assessment: (invent); diagnosis: Voice Disorder (Inadequate Loudness); referred by Dr. Melanie Mallard, Otolaryngologist

Identifying information

Arrange appropriately

(L1H)

BACKGROUND AND REASONS FOR REFERRAL

Who, how old a person, referred when, to which clinic and why?

Use the information above

No prior assessment

Informant: Self

Summarize the history of the voice disorder.

Client reports that: his voice is too soft for his occupation (high school teacher); voice gets tired too soon during the working days; students complain because of too soft voice; has had the problem for the past 2 years; not much variation

Write your report. Invent information as needed.

(L1H)
Write the name and address of the clinic.

(L1H)
What kind of report?

Identifying information

Arrange appropriately

Write the L1H that goes here.

Indent paragraphs.

When, who, and how old a person was referred to which clinic and why?

Summarize the voice disorder.

Data Sheet

HISTORY	**(L1H)**
Birth and Development	**(L2H)**
No relevant information; eliminate this heading in the report	Prenatal, birth Mother's health Early development Early language development
Medical History	**(L2H)**
ENT report negative; normal laryngeal structures No medical basis for the symptoms voice treatment recommended	Diseases of significance

Write your report. Invent information as needed.

(L1H)

(L2H)

Prenatal, birth

Mother's health

Early development

(L2H)

Medical history

Diseases of

significance

Data Sheet	
Family, Social, and Educational History	**(L2H)**
The only son	Family How many children?
No history of communicative disorder	Any family history of communicative problems?
Mother: college graduate; a college counselor Father: college graduate; a college admissions officer	Parents' education and occupation

Write your report. Invent information as needed.

(L2H)

Family
How many children?

Any family history of
communicative
problems?

Parents' education and
occupation

Data Sheet	
ASSESSMENT INFORMATION	**(L1H)**
Orofacial Examination	**(L2H)**
	Describe the orofacial examination: integrity of oral and facial structures.
Negative	
Hearing Screening	**(L2H)**
Screened: 250, 500, 1000, 2000, 4000, and 8000 Hz at 25 dBHL	What frequencies were screened and at what level?
Passed	What were the results?

Write your report. Invent information as needed.

(L1H)

(L2H)

Describe the orofacial examination:
Integrity of oral and facial structures.

(L2H)

What frequencies were screened and at what level?

What were the results?

Data Sheet

Speech, Language, and Fluency

Based on the observation of conversational speech during interview, judged to be within normal limits

Speech 100% intelligible

(L2H)

How were they assessed?

What was the speech intelligibility?

Write your report. Invent information as needed.

(L2H)

How were they assessed?

What were the results?

What was the speech intelligibility?

Data Sheet

Voice   (L2H)

Subjectively rated on a 5-point scale from very soft to very loud   How was voice
Received a rating of 2, soft voice   assessed?
Also measured with a sound level meter with the microphone placed at 8
inches from the client's face
Measurement showed 68 dB, judged too soft   What were the results?
Additional data: in each class period, the client's students request some
five to six times to speak louder
Was asked to baserate the frequency with which the students request him
to speak louder over 5 consecutive days

Data Sheet

Write your report. Invent information as needed.

(L2H)

How was voice assessed?

What were the results of the analysis?

Data Sheet

DIAGNOSTIC SUMMARY	**(L1H)**
Clinical judgment and instrumental measurement suggest too soft voice that cannot meet the demands of the client's social and occupational life	Summarize the voice disorder.
A significant occupational handicap	

DIAGNOSTIC SUMMARY

Clinical judgment and instrumental measurement suggest too soft voice that cannot meet the demands of the client's social and occupational life A significant occupational handicap

(L1H)
Summarize the voice disorder.

RECOMMENDATIONS

(L1H)
Do you recommend treatment?
What are the priority treatment targets?

Treatment recommended

Shape a louder voice considered appropriate for classroom teaching

Reduce or eliminate the number of student requests to speak louder by shaping appropriately louder voice

Who submitted the report?
Write the name, degree, and title.

Submitted by_____ (Your name)

Who approved the report?
Write the name, degree, certification, and title.

Approved by _____ (Clinical supervisor)

Write your report. Invent information as needed

(L1H)

Summarize the voice disorder.

(L1H)

Do you recommend treatment?

What are the priority treatment targets?

Who submitted the report?

Write the name, degree, and title.

Who approved the report?

Write the name, degree, certification, and title.

Note to Student Clinicians

Contact your clinic secretary for additional examples of assessment reports. Take note of variations in formats. Practice writing reports according to your clinic format. Use the practice formats presented in this section.

C.1.6. REPORTS WRITTEN AS LETTERS TO A REFERRING PROFESSIONAL

In many settings, especially in private speech and hearing clinics, a diagnostic report may be written as a letter to a referring professional. For instance, a physician might refer a man with laryngectomy to a speech-language pathologist who then writes a letter to the physician and summarizes the assessment information.

Another reason to write an assessment report in the form of a letter is to make a referral to a specialist whose recommendation is needed before treatment may be started . For instance, a woman with a hoarse voice might first go to a speech clinic. The clinician who evaluates her should write a letter to a laryngologist summarizing her assessment results and referring the client for a laryngeal examination. Treatment is begun only after the laryngeal examination does not contraindicate voice therapy.

Assessment reports written in the form of a letter to a referring professional contain only the most important factors. It is assumed that the professional who has referred the client to you has on file all the details about the patient. Therefore, the speech-language clinician need not write about the client's personal, family, and medical history. Instead, the clinician will limit the report to the most essential elements of his or her assessment and recommendations. However, the letter that makes a referral to another professional after an assessment may contain additional information about the client and his or her history of the communicative problem. Two examples follow.

SIERA SPEECH AND HEARING CENTER
JOHNSONVILLE, WYOMING
SPEECH-LANGUAGE EVALUATION

April 15, 1993

June Johnson, M.D.

Johnson Medical Group

Johnsonville, WY

RE: Victor Valence

Dear Dr. Johnson:

Thank you for referring Mr. Victor Valence, a 72 year–old male, for a speech-language assessment. I saw Mr. Valence at our clinic for a speech evaluation and consultation on April 12, 1993. I understand that Mr. Valence was diagnosed with throat cancer approximately 3 years ago. At that time, he received radiation therapy. Because this treatment was not successful in controlling his cancer, Mr. Valence underwent a total laryngectomy on December 1992.

His wife accompanied him to the session. Mr. and Mrs. Valence both have significant hearing losses. Mr. Valence owns a hearing aid which he does not wear. Since his laryngectomy, Mr. Valence has been communicating through the use of writing and gesture. No feeding or swallowing problems were reported.

ORAL-PERIPHERAL EXAMINATION

An oral-peripheral examination revealed adequate functioning for the production of speech sounds. Diadochokinetic rates were within normal limits. Mr. Valence's cannula had been removed and his stoma appeared to be healing well.

ELECTRONIC SPEECH DEVICES

Several electronic speech devices were available for Mr. Valence to see and try. These devices included: the Cooper Rand Intra-Oral Electrolarynx, the Romet Electrolarynx, the Western Electric Electrolarynx, the Aurex/Neovox Electrolarynx, and the Servox Electrolarynx (neck devices). Mr. Valence was no longer experiencing tenderness and pain in the neck area, so a neck device was utilized. Instructions were provided on the placement of the Aurex and on compensatory articulation strategies needed to use it. Mr. Valence was then given this electronic larynx to use at home until one of his own could be ordered or purchased. He was told to place the electrolarynx on his cheek if he experienced any neck pain or tenderness. In addition, forms were completed to obtain a free electrolarynx from the phone company to be used as a back-up device in the future.

ESOPHAGEAL SPEECH

The altered anatomy and physiology of the pharynx, trachea, and esophagus, and their relationship to the production of speech sounds were discussed and visually demonstrated for Mr. Valence. Esophageal speech sound production was then attempted using the following air intake methods: injection, inhalation, and plosive injection. Mr. Valence was successful in producing sound via the consonant injection and plosive injection methods. He could produce a variety of syllables and words.

TRACHEO-ESOPHAGEAL PUNCTURE

Because you had suggested the possibility of a tracheo-esophageal (TE) puncture to Mr. Valence, I discussed this procedure in detail. Using pictures and drawings, I explained the surgical procedure. I showed Mr. Valence samples of various prostheses and discussed with him procedures for care and management of the TE puncture and prosthesis. Mr. and Mrs. Valence were both enthusiastic about this speech option. In my opinion, Mr. Valence's relatively good health, dexterity, motivation, independence in caring for his stoma, ability to produce esophageal phonation, and favorable disposition toward this procedure make him an excellent candidate. In addition, the size, location, and shape of his stoma are consistent with successful placement of a TE puncture.

ADDITIONAL INFORMATION

I gave Mr. Valence information on ordering such supplies as stoma covers, filters, dickies, and mock turtleneck shirts. I also told him about the "Lost Chord Club" and the support he and his wife might receive from the club.

SUMMARY AND RECOMMENDATION

Mr. Valence was highly motivated to develop a form of verbal communication, primarily through the use of a TE puncture. He also is interested in using an electrolarynx. He demonstrated excellent potential for the use of a TE puncture and good beginning skills for the use of an electronic larynx. Therefore I recommend that Mr. Valence receive speech treatment for a minimum of two times a week for an initial period of 3 months. The treatment will emphasize functional communication through the use of a voice prosthesis (if the TE puncture procedure is done) and an electrolarynx. If a TE puncture is not done, the development of esophageal speech will be pursued.

Thank you for referring this patient to our center. Please contact me if you have questions or comments.

Yours sincerely,

Francine Maxtor, M.A., CCC-SP
Speech-Language Pathologist

NORTHEAST SPEECH AND HEARING CENTER
Albany, New York

March 10, 1993

Bart Barkley, MD

Albany Medical Associates

RE: Mrs. Zenner Zantosh

Dear Dr. Barkley:

I saw Mrs. Zantosh, a 58–year–old female, on March 5, 1992 for an assessment of her voice. The presenting complaints were hoarseness and weakness of the voice, especially when singing. The onset of her dysphonia was approximately 2 years ago, however, her voice production deteriorated in January, 1993. An indirect laryngoscopy on February 17, 1992 was negative. Mrs. Zantosh, who has recently moved to Albany, has sought treatment for her persistent dysphonia.

HISTORY

Mrs. Zantosh reports a history of chronic laryngitis secondary to smoking. Eighteen years ago, Mrs. Zantosh was diagnosed as having leukoplakia and quit smoking at that time. History is negative for alcoholic beverage consumption. Mrs. Zantosh reportedly drinks two to three cups of coffee daily, eats spicy foods, uses salt frequently, and eats dairy products occasionally. Mrs. Zantosh related that she drinks approximately two to three glasses of water each day.

Mrs. Zantosh takes Seldane BID for her allergies and periodically has post-nasal drainage. Additional prescription drugs which have been prescribed include Synthroid and Naprosin. She reports hypothyroidism and tonsillectomy in childhood. Mrs. Zantosh states that her most recent case of laryngitis was in May 1992. Previous audiometric testing indicated a mild to moderate hearing loss in her left ear, which was identified approximately 3 years ago.

Mrs. Zantosh is employed as a teacher at McLane High School and also taught chorus at the school. Her history is positive for talking in noise at work and in the car, yelling and cheering, loud and excessive talking over long periods of time, and loud laughter. Telephone usage is reportedly minimal. However, until recently, Mrs. Zantosh sang in choir at church and was involved in group singing performances. Mrs. Zantosh says that she is typically hoarse following singing and has a weak voice when she is trying to sing at the middle and lower registers. She reported that her frustration with her reduced ability to sing has caused her stress.

Because she lives alone, Mrs. Zantosh experiences routine periods of vocal rest. She occasionally uses throat lozenges to alleviate the sensation of a dry throat from singing.

ASSESSMENT INFORMATION

Mrs. Zantosh was responsive and cooperative throughout the evaluation period. The results appeared to be indicative of her typical vocal behavior.

Vocally Abusive Behaviors: During the assesment session, Mrs. Zantosh cleared her throat 16 times. She also exhibited several instances of hard glottal attacks.

Vocal Parameters: Vocal quality was noted to be intermittently harsh, with a low vocal pitch. An elevated loudness level also was evident. Nonetheless, her overall pitch and loudness ranges appeared to be within normal limits during assessment. Mrs. Zantosh occasionally produced pitch breaks and exhibited vocal fry at the ends of her sentences. A deterioration in her voice was noted across an oral reading passage. She was able to prolong the /s/ sound for 31 seconds and prolonged /z/ for 38 seconds. Both of these results were within normal limits.

Physical Parameters: Mrs. Zantosh maintained a forward head position during the evaluation. Additionally, she complained of tension in her shoulders. Oral mobility was considered to be good.

Trial Therapy: Mrs. Zantosh was able to produce a clear voice following the clinician's instructions to raise her pitch. With modeling, she also could exhibit gentle phonatory onset.

Oral-Peripheral Exam: An inspection of the patient's oral-facial complex revealed structures and functions to be within normal limits.

SUMMARY AND RECOMMENDATIONS

Mrs. Zantosh presents a clinically significant voice disorder, characterized by a harsh quality, low pitch, and reportedly increased vocal loudness. Additionally, she engages in several vocally abusive behaviors. It is recommended that she receive intensive voice therapy on a twice-a-week basis for a period of approximately 3 months. Her prognosis for improvement is considered good. Because her role as a teacher places such demands on voice production, it is vital that she receive voice therapy at this time to improve her voice and to prevent any further deterioration in her vocal skills.

The following treatment objectives seem appropriate:

1.   Train Mrs. Zantosh to produce a clear vocal quality at a conversational level across persons, settings, and situations.

2.   Increase vocal pitch.

3.   Reduce loudness during conversation.

4.   Eliminate pitch breaks and vocal fry.

5.   Improve head positioning during speech.

6.   Establish a vocal hygiene program.

I am referring Mrs. Zantosh to you for a medical examination prior to initiating voice treatment.   If you have questions or suggestions about the proposed plan of treatment, please contact me.

Yours sincerely,

_____

Janet Jackson, Ph.D., CCC-SP
Speech-Language Pathologist

Note to Student Clinicians

Find out the format and content of letters your clinic may send to insurance companies, government agencies, and private organizations that fund speech, language, and hearing services. Some of these offices may receive printed forms that the clinic fills-out and sends for reimbursement.

C.1.7. PRACTICE IN WRITING REPORTS AS LETTERS

C.1.7. ASSESSMENT REPORT AS A LETTER: *ARTICULATION DISORDER*

On the next page, write a letter to a referring pediatrician summarizing your assessment of a child with an articulation disorder

Data Sheet	
Your Clinic's name and address (invent)	**(L1H)** Use the standard letter format
Date	
The pediatrician's name and address (invent)	
RE: The child's name (invent)	
Salutation:	
Use the following information to construct a letter	Brief history
No need to use headings or subheadings	
Child, 8 years old	
Mother brought the child to the clinic	
No significant medical, prenatal, natal, or developmental history of significance to speech	
Has an older brother and a younger sister (invent their ages)	
No family history of communicative disorders	
Doing well in school	
Negative orofacial examination	Orofacial examination

Write your letter. Invent information as needed.

(L1H)

Use the standard letter format

Brief history

Orofacial examination

Data Sheet	
Goldman-Fristeo Test of Articulation Conversational speech sample omissions and substitutions (invent)	Assessment methods and results
No language, voice, or fluency problems (informally assessed during the interview)	Comments on other aspects of communication
Treatment is recommended Suggest the treatment goals	Treatment information
Thank you, call me and so forth	Concluding remarks
Type your name Sign your name	Your name, degree, and signature

Write your letter. Invent information as needed.

Assessment methods
and results

Comments on other
aspects of
communication

Treatment information

Concluding remarks

Your name, degree,
and signature

Note to Student Clinicians

Think of other kinds of letters clinicians might write. Contact your clinic director to find out what kinds of letters are routinely sent out by the clinic.

C.2. TREATMENT PLANS

The treatment plans written for clients vary across professional settings. The plans written in university clinics are perhaps more detailed than those written at other settings. A student who learns to write detailed and comprehensive treatment plans can easily write less extensive and briefer reports. Examples of more and less detailed treatment plans follow.

C.2.1. COMPREHENSIVE TREATMENT PLANS

Some supervisors may ask you to write a comprehensive treatment plan for your client. A comprehensive treatment plan is more detailed than a brief treatment plan, which often is described as a lesson plan. Such a detailed treatment plan includes the following components:

1. A brief summary of previous assessment data
2. Treatment targets
3. Treatment and probe procedures
4. Maintenance program
5. Follow-up and booster treatment procedures

A student who writes a comprehensive treatment plan understands the total management program for a client. The student may or may not complete the program in a semester or quarter. Nonetheless, writing a comprehensive treatment program is a good exercise in visualizing the entire treatment sequence from the beginning to the end.

C.2.2. COMPREHENSIVE TREATMENT PLAN: *ARTICULATION DISORDER*

UNIVERSITY SPEECH AND HEARING CLINIC

TREATMENT PLAN

Name: Oliver Driver   Date of Birth: February 1, 1986
Address: 312 N. South #111   File no.: 900111-3
City: Martinsville, 64812   Diagnosis: Articulation Disorder
Telephone: 782-9832   Semesters in Therapy: 1
School: University Preschool   Date of Report: June 19, 1990

BACKGROUND INFORMATION

Oliver Driver, a 4-year-old male, began his first semester of speech treatment at the University Speech and Hearing Clinic on February, 1990. Oliver's speech and language were evaluated on January 15, 1990. The evaluation revealed an articulation disorder characterized by substitutions, omissions, and reduced intelligibility. See his folder for a diagnostic report. Treatment was recommended to train correct production of misarticulated phonemes to increase speech intelligibility.

TARGET BEHAVIORS

Based on inconsistent production during assessment, the following phonemes was selected for the initial treatment: /p/, /m/, /s/, /k/, and /g/. Production of each phoneme was baserated with 20 stimulus words administered on modeled and evoked discrete trials. Oliver's correct production of the target phonemes on modeled and evoked baserate trials were as follows:

/p/: 15%
/m/: 10%
/s/: 22%
/k/: 18%
/g/: 14%

Treatment was begun after obtaining the baserates. The following general treatment procedures will be used during the semester. The procedures will be modified as suggested by Oliver's performance data. These changes will be described in the final summary report.

TREATMENT AND PROBE PROCEDURES

Training for each target phoneme will begin at the word level. When Oliver's probe response rate at the word level meets a 90% correct criterion, training will be initiated on two-word phrases. A similar probe criterion will be used to shift training to sentences and then to conversational speech.

Intermixed probes on which trained and untrained words, phrases, or sentences are alternated will be administered every time Oliver meets a tentative training criterion of 90% correct response rate on a block of 20 evoked training trials. Oliver will be trained to meet this criterion at each level of response topography (words, phrases, sentences).

Initially, the clinician will provide stimulus pictures, but Oliver will be required to find at least five pictures in magazines or draw two pictures representing the target sound and bring them to the clinic sessions. After he correctly produces the target sound on five consecutive trials, he will paste the pictures in a book to be used for both clinic and home practice.

Training will begin at each level with discrete trials and modeling. The clinician will show Oliver a picture, ask a question ("What is this?") and model the response (word or phrase). Oliver will then be required to imitate the clinician's production. When Oliver correctly imitates the target sound on five consecutive trials, modeling will be discontinued. The clinician will show Oliver a picture and ask "What is this?" to evoke a response.

At the modeled and evoked word levels, verbal reinforcement will be administered on an FR1 schedule for correct productions. At the phrase and sentence levels, a FR4 will be used. At the conversational level, verbal reinforcement will be delivered on an approximate VR5 schedule. All incorrect productions at each level will immediately be interrupted by saying "stop."

Modeling will be reintroduced if Oliver gives two to four incorrect responses on the evoked trials. Shaping with manual guidance will be used as necessary.

All productions will be charted by the clinician. Oliver also will chart productions with an X under the *happy face* or X under the *sad face*. At the end of each session, Oliver will assist the clinician in recording his progress on a graph.

It is expected that different target sounds will reach the training criterion at different times. Therefore, the clinician expects to train several sounds at different response topographies in each session. Some sounds may be trained at the word level while others may be trained at the phrase or even sentence level. When the initially selected target sounds meet the criterion of 90% correct probe rate in conversational speech in the clinic, new target sounds will be baserated and trained.

MAINTENANCE PROGRAM

After Oliver produces the target sound with 90% accuracy at the evoked word level, his mother will be asked to participate in treatment. Initially, she will observe the treatment procedure, and she will present stimulus items and chart correct and incorrect productions. She will be trained to immediately reinforce the correct productions and stopping Oliver at the earliest sign of an inaccurate production.

After Oliver's mother identifies correct and incorrect responses with at least 90% accuracy in the clinic session, she will be trained to work with him at home. The mother will begin with such structured activities as reciting from a list or "reading" from the book he is developing in treatment. Assignments will progress to monitoring and recording speech during dinner and phone conversations with Oliver's grandmother. She will be trained to prompt and then praise the correct productions in conversational speech. Oliver, the clinician, and Oliver's mother will review tape-recorded home assignments. The mother will be given feedback on the procedures implemented at home.

When Oliver produces the target sound with 90% accuracy in conversation in the sessions, he will be taken out of the clinic to practice correct productions in nonclinical situations. The clinician will take Oliver for a walk on campus and talk with him. Subsequently, he may be taken to the campus bookstore, library, cafeteria, and other places. Eventually, his speech may be monitored informally in shopping centers and restaurants.

When Oliver's speech is 98% intelligible and he produces most of his speech sounds at least 90% correct, he may be dismissed from treatment. A follow-up visit will be scheduled for 6 months after dismissal. Based on the initial follow-up results, booster treatment, treatment for persistent errors, or additional follow-up assessments will be planned.

Submitted by: _____

       Marla Model, B.A.

       Student Clinician

Approved by: _____

       Barbara Sierra, M.S., CCC/SP

       Clinical Supervisor

C.2.2. BRIEF TREATMENT PLANS

Brief or short-term treatment plans, also known as lesson plans, are probably used more frequently. The scope of these plans varies across clinics and supervisors. Some plans describe what will be done in only a session or two. Others might describe treatment objectives and procedures planned for a week, a quarter, or a semester. Even those plans that describe the plan for a semester may not be as comprehensive as a complete treatment plan. In some plans, only the treatment objectives may be listed. However, all treatment plans—long or short—should contain a statement of prognosis and a description of target behaviors, treatment procedures, and performance criteria.

The examples of brief treatment plans given on the following pages show slightly different formats in which they may be written. The sampling of formats is not comprehensive; the examples suggest a few basic variations.

C.2.2. BRIEF TREATMENT PLAN: *FLUENCY DISORDER*

SPEECH AND HEARING CLINIC
EASTERN STATE UNIVERSITY
BEDFORD, CALIFORNIA

James Foxx, a 23-year-old male, was seen on February 2, 1993 for a speech evaluation at the Speech and Hearing Clinic of Eastern State University, Bedford, California. The results of the evaluation indicate a severe fluency disorder with 21% dysfluency rate in conversational speech. His dysfluencies are characterized by repetitions, prolongations, pauses, interjections, and revisions. A fluency treatment program was recommended. With consistent treatment, prognosis for improved fluency was judged to be good.

The following treatment program has been developed for James.

Final Treatment Objective: A dysfluency rate that does not exceed 5% in James's home and other nonclinical settings.

TARGET BEHAVIORS

1. **Appropriate management of airflow.** To produce and sustain fluency in conversational speech, James will be taught to inhale and then immediately exhale a slight amount of air before phonation. He also will be taught to sustain a smooth airflow throughout his utterances.

2. **Gentle onset of phonation.** James will be taught to initiate phonation in a soft and easy manner.

3. **Reduced speech rate.** James will be taught to prolong vowels to reduce his speech rate and to achieve continuous phonation.

4. **Continuous phnation.** Thougout an utterance, James will be taught to maintain continuous phonation by not pausing between words.

TREATMENT PROCEDURES

1. A baseline of dysfluency rates in conversational speech will be established before starting the treatment.

2. Treatment will begin at the phrase or short sentence level.

3. As James sustains 98% fluency at each level of response complexity, utterance length will be increased.

4. The clinician will verbally reinforce the production of all target behaviors including the resulting fluency.

5. The clinician will give corrective feedback for incorrect responses, including dysfluencies.

6. As James sustains 98% fluency in conversational speech, maintenance procedures will be implemented. James's wife and a colleague of his will be trained in evoking and reinforcing skills of fluency. The clinician will take James to extraclinical situations to evoke and reinforce his fluency skills.

7. Follow-up and booster treatment will be arranged as needed.

Signed:_____

      Gloria Marquez, B.A.

      Student Clinician

Signed:_____

      Henriette Borden, Ph.D., CCC-SP

      Speech-Language Pathologist, Supervisor

I understand the results of the evaluation and agree to the recommended treatment plan.

Signed:_____   Date:_____

James Foxx

C.2.2 BRIEF TREATMENT PLAN: *ARTICULATION DISORDER*

VALLEY SPEECH AND HEARING CENTER
NORDSTROM, MAINE

Rudy Amos, a 7-year-old boy was referred to the Valley Speech and Hearing Center for assessment and treatment of an articulation disorder. According to an assessment made on February 10, 1993 Rudy has an articulation disorder limited to omissions of the following phonemes in both the word initial and final positions: /k, l, s, t, r/, and /z/. Treatment was recommended, and prognosis for improvement was judged to be excellent because Rudy was readily stimulable and highly cooperative during a brief period of trial therapy.

The treatment was begun on February 15, 1983. A baseline suggested 0 to 10% accuracy on the target phonemes.

The treatment will have the following objectives and procedures.

Objective 1. Correct production of misarticulated phonemes in the initial position of 10 probe (untrained) words at a minimum of 90% accuracy.

Procedure: Pictures that help evoke words with the target sounds in the initial position will be used. All correct responses will be modeled and verbally reinforced. Corrective feedback will be given for incorrect responses.

Objective 2. Correct production of misarticulated phonemes in the final position of 10 probe (untrained) words at a minimum of 90% accuracy.

Procedures: Pictures that help evoke words with the target sounds in the final position will be used. All correct responses will be modeled and verbally reinforced. Corrective feedback will be given for incorrect responses.

Objective 3. Correct production of misarticulated phonemes in 20 probe phrases and 20 probe sentences.

Procedure: Picture description and controlled conversation will be used to evoke target utterances containing the misarticulated phonemes. Modeling will be provided as needed. Correct responses will be reinforced on a variable schedule designed to progressively reduce the amount of feedback. Corrective feedback will be given for all incorrect responses.

Objective 4. Correct production of misarticulated phonemes in conversational speech with varied audience. Initially, the clinician will evoke the conversational speech. When Rudy's accuracy of production in conversational speech reaches at least 80%, other persons will serve as the audience.

Objective 5. Training Rudy's mother to evoke and reinforce correct productions in conversational speech at home.

Procedure: The mother will be asked to initially observe the sessions and later participate in the treatment sessions. She will be trained in recognizing the correct productions and in immediately praising Rudy. Taped home speech samples will be used to asses the correct production of phonemes at home.

The dismissal criterion: A 90% or better correct production of the target phonemes in conversational speech produced in extraclinical situations.

The procedure will be modified as found necessary during the treatment sessions.

Signed _____

       Mohamed Ali, M.A., CCC-SP

       Speech-Language Pathologist

I understand the treatment program, and I agree to it.

Signed _____

       Mrs. Lydia Amos

       Mother

C.2.2. BRIEF TREATMENT PLAN: *LANGUAGE DISORDER*

SPEECH AND HEARING CLINIC
SOUTHERN STATE UNIVERSITY
JOHNSTONVILLE, LOUISIANA

Timothy Krebs, a 4-year-old boy was evaluated at the Speech and Hearing Clinic at the Southern State University on February 7, 1993. The evaluation revealed a severe language disorder. Case history and assessment data showed that his language performance is limited to a few words and phrases. A detailed assessment report can be found in Timothy's file. A language treatment program was recommended.

Timothy will be seen two times weekly in sessions lasting 45 min. His mother will accompany him to the clinic and will participate in treatment sessions. It is judged that prognosis for improved language performance is good provided that the treatment is consistent and that a home treatment and maintenance program can be sustained. The following treatment objectives were selected for this semester (Spring, 1993).

INITIAL TREATMENT OBJECTIVES

With the help of Timothy's mother, the following 20 targets consisting of single words or two-word phrases of high functional value were selected for initial treatment:

cup	sock	milk	shoe	Jenny (sister)
juice	more	eat	give me	walking
no more	I want	cookie	candy	bath
shirt	look!	Hi	Binny (dog)	John (friend)

SUBSEQUENT TREATMENT OBJECTIVES

Additional vocabulary items

Expansion of single words into two word phrases and sentences

Early morphological features (present progressive, regular plural, possessive, prepositions, pronouns, etc.)

INITIAL TREATMENT PROCEDURES

1. Pictures, objects, acted-out situations, and role-playing will be used as stimuli to evoke the target words or phrases.

2. The clinician and the mother will take turns in evoking the target words or phrases.

3. Initially, gross approximations will be reinforced by verbal praise and such natural reinforcers as handing an object, complying with a request, and so forth. Subsequently, only better approximations will be reinforced.

4. All correct and incorrect productions will be measured.

5. Responses that are produced with 90% accuracy across two sessions will be expanded into longer phrases or simple sentences.

6. The mother will be asked to conduct similar treatment sessions at home and bring taped samples of sessions for evaluation and feedback.

It is expected that Timothy will need extended treatment and that both the treatment objectives and procedures will be modified in light of his performance data.

Signed:_____

   Trisha Muniz, B.A.

   Student Clinician

I understand the results of the evaluation and agree to the recommended treatment plan.

Signed:_____

   Client, Parent, or Guardian

Signed:_____

   Maya Real, M.A., CCC-SP

   Speech-Language Pathologist and Clinical Supervisor

Date_____

C.2.2. BRIEF TREATMENT PLAN: *VOICE DISORDER*

THE SUNSHINE SPEECH AND HEARING CENTER
ZINGSVILLE, VERMONT

Roshana Hersh, a 21-year-old female college student was seen at the Sunshine Speech and Hearing Center on March 10, 1993 for a voice evaluation. The evaluation suggested a pattern of vocal abuse associated with a persistent hoarseness of voice, low pitch, and socially inappropriate intensity. Her vocal abuse consists mainly of excessive talking over the phone and shouting at children she supervises as a teacher's aid in a kindergarten school. The detailed case history and assessment data can be found in her file. A treatment program to improve her voice quality was recommended. Considering her high degree of motivation for improvement that she expressed during the interview, prognosis was judged to be good.

Treatment Targets

Goal 1: Production of clear voice at least 90% of the time Roshana speaks by reducing the hoarseness of voice

    Objective 1a. Reduced amount of talking over the phone.

    Objective 1b. Reduced amount of shouting at the school.

Goal 2. Increased vocal pitch

    Objective 2a. Higher pitch at the level of words and phrases.

    Objective 2b. Higher pitch at the level of conversational speech.

Goal 3. Decreased vocal intensity

    Objective 3a. Softer voice at the level of words and phrases.

    Objective 3b. Softer voice at the level of conversational speech.

Treatment Procedures

Objectives 1a and 1b. During the first week, the durations of Roshana's telephone conversation will be baserated. She will be asked to keep a diary and record the duration of each telephone conversation. During the second week, Roshana will be asked to reduce by 10% the amount of telephone conversation time. She will continue to record the amount of time she spends talking. In subsequent weeks, she will be asked to progressively decrease the amount of time spent on telephone until the duration is reduced by about 50%.

The frequency of shouting also will be similarly baserated. Roshana will then be asked to reduce the frequency of shouting behavior in 10% decrements until the frequency approaches zero.

Objectives 2a and 2b. The Visi-Pitch will be used to shape a higher pitch consistent with Roshana's gender and age. The treatment will start at the word and phrase level and move to conversational speech level.

Objectives 3a and 3b. The Visi-Pitch will be used to progressively decrease the vocal intensity until it is clinically judged to be appropriate for Roshana. The treatment will start at the word and phrase level and move to conversational speech level.

A maintenance program which includes an analysis of speech samples from home and periodic follow-up and booster treatment will be implemented.

Signed:_____

Pero Boss, B.A.

Student Clinician

I understand the results of the evaluation and agree to the recommended treatment plan.

Signed:_____

Roshana Hersh

Client

Signed:_____

Moss Nero, M.A., CCC-SP

Speech-Language Pathologist and Clinical Supervisor

Date_____

C.2.3. INDIVIDUALIZED EDUCATIONAL PROGRAMS

In public schools, clinicians are required by law to develop individualized educational programs. Clinicians in a typical university or hospital speech and hearing clinic do the same. Individual treatment plans described so far are comparable to individualized educational programs.

Clinicians often do not have time to write lengthy or narrative treatment plans for the children they serve. Therefore, most public school clinicians use printed forms to select treatment targets for the children they treat. Formats vary across school districts, some being more detailed than others. In this section, a few examples of printed individualized education plans for speech-language services are provided.

CENTRAL COAST UNIFIED SCHOOL DISTRICT
INDIVIDUALIZED EDUCATIONAL PLAN FOR SPEECH AND LANGUAGE SERVICES

Oral Language and Verbal Expression

Student's Name_____   Birthdate_____

School_____ Grade_____ Date_____

Speech-Language Pathologist_____

Criteria for Placement: _____

Goal: To improve oral language and verbal expression

Present Level of Performance: *See assessment report*	Target Date	Met On (Date)	Not Met
Objectives: By <u>6/93</u> the student will complete the following objectives with 90% accuracy as measured by pre- and posttests, specialists observation, client-specific procedures, or other procedures (specify): _____ _____			
Improve Oral Language through:			
Social Interaction with others: (Check the targets selected)			
1. __✔ verbally respond when spoken to	12/92		
2. __✔ verbally express feelings and needs	2/93		
3. __ give personal information upon request			
4. __✔ ask and answer questions	4/93		
5. __ initiate conversation			
6. __ share personal experiences			
7. __✔ describe events in detail	5/93		
8. __ report factual information			
9. __ interact verbally with others			
10. __ give sequential, accurate verbal directions			
11.__✔ take part in class discussions and reports			
12. __ other _____	6/93		

ATLANTIC UNIFIED SCHOOL DISTRICT
LANGUAGE, SPEECH, AND HEARING
INDIVIDUALIZED EDUCATIONAL PROGRAM OBJECTIVES
Treatment of Articulation

Pupil _____   Speech-Language and Hearing Specialist

Date _____   _____

School_____   Services started on _____

Goal: Improved intelligibility of speech through correct production of phonemes at 90% accuracy.

Target Date	Objectives (Check the ones selected)	Evaluation and Treatment Procedures	Date Objectives Met
	Articulation		
	Correct production of the following phonemes: /d/, /t/, /p/, /ʒ/, and /l/	Paired stimuli method of treatment	
10/92	__✔ in isolation	Probes to assess production in untrained contexts	10/92
10/92	__✔ in syllables		10/92
11/92	__✔ in words		11/92
12/92	__✔ initial		12/92
1/93	__✔ medial		1/93
	__✔ final		
	__✔ in phrases		
2/93	__✔ in sentences		2/93
3/93	__✔ conversational speech		4/93
5/93	__✔ in natural settings		6/93
6/93	__✔ other		not met
6/93			not met
	increased intelligibility		partially met by 6/93

GULF COAST UNIFIED SCHOOL DISTRICT
DEPARTMENT OF SPECIAL EDUCATIONAL SERVICES
LANGUAGE, SPEECH, AND HEARING
INDIVIDUALIZED EDUCATIONAL PROGRAMS
Treatment of Voice Disorders

Student's Name: _____ Speech-Language and Hearing Specialist

_____

School: _____   Date _____

Program initiation date_____

Goal: By _3/93_ the student will complete the following objectives with 80% accuracy.

Target Date	Objectives (Check the Ones Selected)	Evaluation and Treatment Procedures	Target Met On (Date)
	Voice Overall Objective: Improved voice quality and appropriate use of voice		
12/92 12/92 1/93	**Pitch** __✔ lower __ higher __ in school __ in other settings	Successive approximation with the help of Visi-Pitch	12/92 12/92 1/93
2/93 2/93 3/93	**Intensity** __ lower (softer voice) __✔ higher (louder voice) __ in school __ in other settings	Conversational probes to assess generalization and maintenance	
	Nasal resonance ___ decrease ___ increase		
	Voice quality ___ reduce hoarseness ___ reduce harshness ___ reduce breathiness Other voice objectives (specify):		

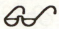

NORTH CENTRAL UNIFIED SCHOOL DISTRICT
SPEECH, LANGUAGE, AND HEARING SERVICES
INDIVIDUALIZED EDUCATIONAL PLAN

Treatment of Fluency Disorders

Student's Name: _____ Speech-Language and Hearing Specialist

_____

School: _____   Date _____

Treatment began on:_____

Goal: Improved fluency in conversational speech produced in extraclinical settings with a dysfluency rate under 5%.

Target Date	Objectives (Check the ones selected)	Evaluation and Treatment Procedures	Objectives Met On
	Fluency		
11/92 12/93 3/93 6/93	Target Skills: __✓ Appropriate management of airflow __✓ Gentle phonatory onset __✓ Reduced rate of speech __✓ in words and phrases __✓ in sentences __✓ in conversational speech __✓ in extraclinical situations. ____ Normal prosody and fluency	Teaching fluency skills with modeling, successive approximation, and verbal reinforcement. fading the slow rate; shaping normal prosody Conversational probes to assess generalization to and maintenance of fluency in clinical and extraclinical situations	11/92 12/93 3/93 Not met Not met

Note to Student Clinicians

Contact the coordinator of speech-language and hearing services in one of the school districts in your area to learn more about variations in individualized educational plans written for students. Before you begin your clinical internships in a public school, practice writing individualized educational plans according to the format accepted in the school.

C.3. PRACTICE IN WRITING TREATMENT PLANS

C.3. COMPREHENSIVE TREATMENT PLAN: *LANGUAGE DISORDERS*

UNIVERSITY SPEECH AND HEARING CENTER
PAN PACIFIC UNIVERSITY
PACIFIC, CALIFORNIA

Data Sheet

Harvey Brokert, 6 yrs. Talks in two- to three-word phrases no sentences Treatment was recommended	Who, how old, when, to where referred? What were the results of evaluation? (Summarize the disorder) Was treatment recommended?
Functional language skills with appropriate grammatic and pragmatic structures produced in natural settings	Final Treatment Objective? **(L2H)**
Initial target behaviors: Teaching noun, auxiliary *is* and verb + *ing; prepositions in, on* and *under; and* pronouns *he* and *she*. All taught in the context of simple sentences	Target Behaviors? **(L2H)**

C.3. COMPREHENSIVE TREATMENT PLAN: *LANGUAGE DISORDERS*

UNIVERSITY SPEECH AND HEARING CENTER

PAN PACIFIC UNIVERSITY

PACIFIC, CALIFORNIA

Write your report. Invent information as needed.

Who, how old, when, to where referred?
What were the results of evaluation? (Summarize the disorder.)
Was treatment recommended?

Final Treatment Objective? (L2H)

Target Behaviors? (L2H)

	Treatment Procedures (L1H)
Data Sheet	
Baseline procedure: one set of evoked and one set of modeled trials; 20 stimulus items for each target	Baseline procedures
Discrete trial procedures: show the stimulus, ask a question, model the response, reinforce or give corrective feedback, record the response, re-present the stimulus for the next trial	Various training and probe criteria
Modeling, verbal praise, natural consequences Five consecutively and correctly imitated responses: shift to evoked Two incorrect responses on evoked trials: reinstate modeling	
Training criterion: 10 consecutively correct, nonimitated responses for each target behavior.	
Intermixed probe procedure	
Ninety percent correct probe response rate: shift training to another stimulus item, a more complex response topography, or another target behavior	

Write your report. Invent information as needed.

Treatment Procedures?
(L1H)

Baseline procedure

Various training and
probe criteria

Data Sheet	
	Maintenance Procedures (L1H)
	Maintenance criterion
Correct production of the selected words at 90% accuracy at the clinic (training) and in nonclinical settings (probe)	
Parent training in arranging conditions for and in reinforcing the production of target words	**Training family members and others**
Initially, parents observe sessions Then they learn to present stimulus items Then they learn to reinforce or give corrective feedback An older brother to be trained in reinforcing target responses	
Informal training in nonclinical settings	**Training in informal (more natural) settings**
	Home samples
Recorded home samples for probe analysis	
Training the production of target behaviors in conversational speech	**Conversational speech**
Subtle contingency management	

Write your report. Invent information as needed.

Maintenance Procedures (L1H)

Maintenance criterion

Training family members and others

Training in informal (more natural) settings

Home samples

Conversational speech

Data Sheet	
Need for long-term training and follow-up	Long-term treatment
Additional target behaviors to be selected as found appropriate	Suggest some potential target behaviors
	Signature lines
	Student Clinician
	Supervisor
	Client

Write your report. Invent information as needed.

Long-term treatment

Suggest some potential targets

Signature lines

Student Clinician

Supervisor

Client

C.3. BRIEF TREATMENT PLAN: *FLUENCY DISORDER*

SPEECH AND HEARING CLINIC
EASTERN STATE UNIVERSITY
BEDFORD, CALIFORNIA

Data Sheet	
James Higginbothams, 27 yrs Self-referred Two speech samples; 23% and 25% dysfluency rate in conversational speech (part-word repetitions, sound prolongations, word and phrase interjections, and broken words) Treatment was recommended Prognosis judged to be good because of expressed high motivation for treatment	Who, how old, when, to where referred? What were the results of evaluation? (Summarize the disorder.) Was treatment recommended?
Normal-sounding fluency with no more than 5% dysfluency rate in nonclinical settings.	Final Treatment Objective? **(L2H)**
Initially, inhalation and a slight exhalation, gentle phonatory onset, and reduced rate with prolonged syllables, near zero dysfluency rate; subsequently, normal prosody and fluency.	Target Behaviors? **(L2H)**

C.3. BRIEF TREATMENT PLAN: *FLUENCY DISORDER*

SPEECH AND HEARING CLINIC
EASTERN STATE UNIVERSITY
BEDFORD, CALIFORNIA

Write your report. Invent information as needed.

	Who, how old, when, to where referred? What were the results of evaluation? (Summarize the disorder.) Was treatment recommended?
	Final Treatment Objective? (**L2H**)
	Target Behaviors? (**L2H**)

Data Sheet	
Controlled utterances and conversational speech; modeling and reinforcement; prompts; and other procedures	Treatment Procedures? (L2H)
Progression from words or phrases to conversational speech.	Establishment
Ninety eight percent fluency in the treatment sessions; 95% for speech probes.	Training and probe criteria
Training the significant others in prompting and slowing down the rate and in reinforcing the client. Training self monitoring skills.	Maintenance strategies
Three months, six months, one year, and 2- year follow-up; booster treatment as needed.	Follow-up and booster treatment
	Signature lines
	Student Clinician
	Supervisor
	Client

Write your report. Invent information as needed.	Treatment Procedures? (L2H)
	Establishment
	Training and probe criteria
	Maintenance strategies
	Follow-up and booster treatment
	Signature lines
	Student Clinician
	Supervisor
	Client

C.3. BRIEF TREATMENT PLAN: *ARTICULATION DISORDER*

VALLEY SPEECH AND HEARING CENTER
NORDSTROM, MAINE

Data Sheet	
Beth Hazleton, 9 yrs.	Who, how old, when, to where referred?
Articulation disorder; omissions: (specify four to six phonemes); substitutions: (specify a few).	What were the results of evaluation? (Summarize the disorder.)
Treatment was recommended.	Was treatment recommended?
Ninety percent correct production in conversational speech in extraclinical situations.	Final Treatment Objective? **(L2H)**
Specify the phonemes and the word positions.	Target Behaviors? **(L2H)**

C.3. BRIEF TREATMENT PLAN: *ARTICULATION DISORDER*

VALLEY SPEECH AND HEARING CENTER
NORDSTROM, MAINE

Write your report. Invent information as needed.

Who, how old, when, to where referred?
What were the results of evaluation?
(Summarize the disorder.)
Was treatment recommended?

Final Treatment Objective? **(L2H)**

Target Behaviors? **(L2H)**

Data Sheet	
	Treatment Procedures (L2H)
Discrete trial procedure or other procedures you select	Establishment
Teach production in words, phrases, sentences, conversational speech Modeling, manual guidance, verbal praise, other procedures	
Ninety percent correct and training and probe, or other criteria you select	Training and probe criteria
	Maintenance
Training the parents and siblings in maintenance procedures	Training family members and others
	Signature lines
	Student Clinician
	Supervisor
	Client

Write your report. Invent information as needed.

	Treatment Procedures (L2H)
	Establishment
	Training and probe criteria
	Maintenance
	Training family members and others
	Signature lines
	Student Clinician
	Supervisor
	Client

C.3. BRIEF TREATMENT PLAN: *LANGUAGE DISORDER*

SPEECH AND HEARING CLINIC
SOUTHERN STATE UNIVERSITY
JOHNSTONVILLE, LOUISIANA

Data Sheet	
Harold Ford, 5 yrs. Mentally retarded Says only six to eight words No phrases, no sentences Treatment was recommended	Who, how old, when, to where referred? What were the results of evaluation? (Summarize the disorder.) Was treatment recommended?
Functional language skills with basic sentence structures produced in natural settings	Final Treatment Objective? (L2H)
Initial target behaviors: Teaching 20 functional words to be produced at 90% accuracy at home	Target Behaviors? (L2H)

C.3. BRIEF TREATMENT PLAN: *LANGUAGE DISORDER*

SPEECH AND HEARING CLINIC

SOUTHERN STATE UNIVERSITY

JOHNSTONVILLE, LOUISIANA

Write your report. Invent information as needed.

Who, how old, when, to where referred?
What were the results of evaluation?
(Summarize the disorder.)
Was treatment recommended?

Final Treatment
Objective? **(L2H)**

Target Behaviors?
(L2H)

Data Sheet

Discrete trial procedures; incidental teaching methods; or other procedures you select	Treatment Procedures? **(L2H)**
Modeling, verbal praise, natural consequences	Establishment
Correct production of the selected words at 90% accuracy at the clinic (training) and in nonclinical settings (probe)	Training and probe criteria
Parent training in arranging conditions for and in reinforcing the production of target words	Maintenance
	Training family members and others
	Signature lines
	Student Clinician
	Supervisor
	Client

Write your report. Invent information as needed.

Treatment Procedures?
(L2H)

Establishment

Training and probe
criteria

Maintenance

Training family
members and others

Signature lines

Student Clinician

Supervisor

Client

C.3. BRIEF TREATMENT PLAN: *VOICE DISORDER*

THE SUNSHINE SPEECH AND HEARING CENTER
ZINGSVILLE, VERMONT

Data Sheet	
Thomas Benson, Jr., 28 yrs.	Who, how old, when, to where referred?
High-pitched voice	What were the results of evaluation? (Summarize the disorder.)
Treatment was recommended	Was treatment recommended?
Vocal pitch judged appropriate for age and gender	Final Treatment Objective? **(L2H)**
Lowered pitch level in words, phrases, sentences, and conversational speech	Target Behaviors? **(L2H)**

C.3. BRIEF TREATMENT PLAN: *VOICE DISORDER*

Write your report. Invent information as needed.

Who, how old, when, to where referred?
What were the results of evaluation? (Summarize the disorder.)
Was treatment recommended?

Final Treatment Objective? **(L2H)**

Target Behaviors? **(L2H)**

Data Sheet	
Shaping lower-pitched voice through modeling and verbal feedback Starting with words and progressing to conversational speech Other procedures you select	Treatment Procedures? (L2H) Establishment
Ninety percent accuracy at each level of training Ninety percent probe criterion in natural settings	Training and probe criteria
Self-monitoring skills	Maintenance
Training Ms. Benson in monitoring and reinforcing appropriate pitch at home	Training family members and others
	Signature lines
	Student Clinician
	Supervisor
	Client

Write your report. Invent information as needed.

Treatment Procedures?
(L2H)

Establishment

Training and probe
criteria

Maintenance

Training family
members and others

Signature lines

Student Clinician

Supervisor

Client

Note to Student Clinicians

Clinical supervisors tend to have their own formats for writing treatment plans. Talk to your supervisor before you write treatment plans for your clients.

C.4. PROGRESS REPORTS

Progress reports, also called final summaries, summarize the methods and results of treatment given during a specified period of time. In academic degree programs, progress reports are typically written at the end of a quarter or semester. In some university programs, progress reports also may be known as *final summaries*. In hospitals and private clinics, they are written according to a setting-specific policy. Generally, they are written to support payment for services by insurance companies and government or private agencies. In such cases, they may be written on a monthly basis. Progress reports are written invariably when the clients are dismissed from services.

A progress report students write under clinical practicum or internship is more likely to give such additional information as the number of and duration of sessions and the clock hours of clinical practicum. Such information is not a part of reports professional clinicians write.

Most progress reports are formal documents written for the file. In some settings, especially in hospitals and private clinics, progress reports may be written in the form of a letter to a referring physician or to a funding agency.

C.4. PROGRESS REPORT: TREATMENT OF STUTTERING

UNIVERSITY SPEECH AND HEARING CLINIC
FREEMONT UNIVERSITY
VALLEYVILLE, CALIFORNIA

PROGRESS REPORT

NAME: James Foxx

BIRTHDATE: January 26, 1971

ADDRESS: Graves 312 B

CITY: Valleyville, CA 90710-3342

TELEPHONE NUMBER: 555-3235

FILE NUMBER: RS92019

DIAGNOSIS: Stuttering

DATE OF REPORT: May 10, 1992

PERIOD COVERED: 2/5/92 to 5-6-92

CLINICIAN: Meena Wong

CLINIC SCHEDULE

Session per week:____2____   Clock hrs. of individual therapy:_25 hrs._

Length of session:____1 hr._____   Clock hrs. of group therapy:____0_____

Number of clinic visits:___24___   Total clock hrs. of therapy:_____25_____

James Foxx, a 21-year-old male college student , was enrolled for his first semester of treatment at the University Speech and Hearing Clinic on February 5, 1992. The presenting complaint was stuttering. An assessment done on February 2, 1992 had revealed a conversational dysfluency rate of 21% in the clinic. A home speech sample had revealed a dysfluency rate of 18.6%. He exhibited interjections, pauses, part-word and whole word repetitions, silent and audible prolongations, revisions, and incomplete phrases.

James's treatment was begun on February 5, 1992. An assessment report and a treatment plan may be found in James's folder.

SUMMARY OF TREATMENT

FINAL TREATMENT OBJECTIVE

Maintenance of fluent speech with a dysfluency rate that does not exceed 5% in natural settings.

TREATMENT TARGETS

Fluency skills described in the treatment plan were taught: Appropriate management of airflow, gentle onset of phonation, and reduced rate of speech.

TREATMENT PROCEDURES

In two clinic baseline samples of conversational speech and a home baseline sample, James's dysfluency rates were: 22%, 21%, and 19%.

Initially, James was taught the skills of fluent speech: nasal inhalation, minimal amount of oral exhalation prior to initiation of phonation, easy phonatory onset, and vowel prolongation. Therapy began at the modeled word level and progressed to words, phrases, sentences, and conversational speech in the clinic. At each level, 98% fluency was required. Verbal reinforcement was provided on an FR 1 schedule. Corrective feedback was given for dysfluencies or failure to manage a target behavior. James was then required to correctly repeat his utterance.

After James had progressed to conversational speech, James, along with the clinician, charted dysfluencies and failure to use a target behavior. Periodically, James orally read printed stories and then summarized what he had read. Student observers periodically participated in treatment sessions to engage in conversation with the client.

PROGRESS

Two clinic probes and a home probe were obtained after the client began using the target fluency skills in conversational speech in the clinic (probes #1 and #2). Each probe consisted of 50 utterances sampled from the client's conversational speech. The results were as follows.

Probe #1: 15% dysfluent (Clinic Sample)

Probe #2: 12% dysfluent (Clinic Sample)

Probe #3: 10% dysfluent (Home Sample)

A final conversational speech sample containing 852 words in 102 utterances was obtained in the semester's final treatment session. This sample was obtained through a conversation with a student observer in the absence of the clinician. Results were as follows:

Dysfluency Types	Frequency
Interjections	23
Pauses	17
Part Word Repetitions	1
Whole Word Repetitions	3
Phrase Repetitions	2
Sound Prolongations	20
Silent Prolongations	6
Incomplete Phrases	2
Total Dysfluencies	**74**
Percent Dysfluency Rate	**8.9**

The results show that James's fluency improved over the course of the semester. He was about 21% dysfluent at the beginning of treatment compared to 8.9% dysfluency at the end of the semester.

RECOMMENDATIONS

Although James' dysfluencies have decreased, he continues to exhibit difficulty in consistently managing the target behaviors. Therefore, it is recommended that James Foxx continue to receive treatment next semester. Treatment should focus on the following:

1. Improved management of fluency skills.

2. Generalization and maintenance of fluent speech

Submitted by:_____

           Layang Chan, B.A.

           Student Clinician

Approved by:_____

           Linda Hensley, Ph.D., CCC-SP

           Speech-Language Pathologist and Clinical Supervisor

C.4. PROGRESS REPORT: *TREATMENT OF AN ARTICULATION DISORDER*

SPEECH AND HEARING CENTER
HENRY HIGGINS CHILDREN'S HOSPITAL
BURLINGTON, VERMONT
PROGRESS REPORT

Period Covered: 9/27/92 to 6/13/93

BACKGROUND INFORMATION

Joe Villa, a 6-year and 3-month-old boy, was seen for a speech and language evaluation at the Speech and Hearing Center of the Henry Higgins Children's Hospital on September 24, 1992. Joe has an articulation disorder characterized mostly by omissions of /s/, /t/, /k/, /b/, and /l/ in the initial and final position of words. An articulation treatment program was recommended. He has received treatment for one semester.

The final treatment objective for Joe is to produce the phonemes he omits with 90% accuracy in conversational speech in extraclinical situations. During the current semester, the following specific objectives were targeted.

PROGRESS

Objective 1. Correct production of /s/, /t/, /k/, /b/, and /l/ in word initial positions at 90% accuracy.

Method and Results: The target phoneme production in word initial positions was base rated with 20 words each. Joe's correct response rate ranged from 0 to 10%. Treatment was begun with the discrete trial procedure involving modeling, imitation, successive approximation, and immediate verbal feedback for correct and incorrect responses. Whenever necessary, the tongue positions were shown with the help of a mirror. Each target sound was trained to a criterion of 10 consecutively correct responses. When four words with a target sound met the training criterion, at least 10 probe words were presented to assess generalization.

Joe has met this training objective. In fact, his correct response rate on these phonemes in word initial positions is between 95 and 100%.

Objective 2. Correct production of /s/, /t/, /k/, /b/, and /l/ in word final positions at 90% accuracy.

Methods and Results: The same procedures used to train the phonemes in the word initial positions were used. Joe has met this objective. His correct response rate on the phonemes in word final positions is between 92 and 96%.

Objective 3. Production of the target sounds in phrases and sentences at 90% accuracy in all word positions.

Method and Results: Joe's correct productions were initially reinforced in phrases that were prepared for training. Soon, he was asked to use the target words in sentences he formulated. Later, Joe's conversational speech was monitored to strengthen the correct production of the phonemes. Verbal reinforcement was used on an FR4 schedule.

Joe has met this objective as his correct production of the target phonemes in conversational speech varies between 90 and 95%.

Objective 4. The development and implementation of a home program to maintain the production of his new speech skills at home and other environments at 90% accuracy.

Methods and Results: Joe's parents, who attended most of the treatment sessions, were trained to recognize, prompt, and reinforce the correct production of target sounds. Parents were asked to hold home treatment sessions twice a week and tape-record the sessions. These taped samples were analyzed to give feedback to the parents. Three conversational probes recorded at home has revealed a 90% correct response rate.

Overall, Joe has made excellent progress in producing the targeted sounds. All treatment objective have been met. Therefore, it is recommended that Joe be dismissed from treatment. A follow-up assessment in 3 months is recommended.

_____

Monica Mendoza, M.A., CCC-SP
Speech-Language Pathologist

C.4. PROGRESS REPORT: LANGUAGE TREATMENT

UNIVERSITY SPEECH AND HEARING CENTER
BELLVIEW UNIVERSITY
BELLVIEW, WASHINGTON

Client: William Shakespeare   Date of Birth: January 10, 1986

Period Covered: 2/5 through 5/15, 1993   Clinician: Noah Webster

CLINIC SCHEDULE

Session per week:____2____   Clock hr of individual therapy:_25 hr_

Length of session:____1 hr____   Clock hr of group therapy:_____0_____

Number of clinic visits:__24__   Total clock hr of therapy:_____25_____

William Shakespeare, a 7-year-old boy, was assessed at the University Speech and Hearing Center of Bellview University for a language disorder. The assessment suggested that his language disorder primarily involved some syntactic structures and pragmatic functions. Treatment was recommended. He has received treatment for a semester. Please see his clinic file for a complete treatment program.

SUMMARY OF TREATMENT

William was cooperative in most treatment sessions. The following treatment procedures and objectives were used.

OBJECTIVE 1. ASKING *WH* QUESTIONS

William was taught to ask the following types of *wh* questions:

What do you mean?

What is it?

What are you doing?

What time is it?

What is your name?

Methods and Results: Baserating showed that William typically did not ask the target questions even when the situation demanded them. In a conversational role-playing situation, William was taught to ask the target questions. Conversational situations were created such that questions of the kind targeted would be appropriate. Conversation was manipulated in various ways to prompt the a target question. For example, Willliam was "Do you live in a condo?" and was immediately modeled the correct question for him to imitate: "Ask, what do you mean?" Or, he was shown a picture he did not know anything about and immediately the question "What is it?" was modeled. When William asked an appropriate question, it was correctly answered. These answers and verbal praise for asking appropriate questions were the reinforcers.

William learned to ask the targeted questions in untrained (probe) contexts with 90% accuracy.

OBJECTIVE 2. TOPIC MAINTENANCE

William was taught to maintain a topic of conversation for progressively increasing durations with 90% accuracy.

Methods and Results: Baserating showed that William typically changed the topic in less than a min. He was taught to maintain a topic of conversation for progressively longer durations. One minute increments were used. Starting with a duration of 1min, he was taught to talk about the same topic for a maximum duration of 5 min. Every time he deviated from the topic, he was asked to stop and a prompt to resume the target topic was given. He was periodically praised for continuing on the same topic.

William learned to maintain a topic of conversation for a minimum of 5 min. On certain probe topics, he continued to talk for up to 10 min.

OBJECTIVE 3. CONVERSATIONAL TURN TAKING

William was taught to take appropriate conversational turns with 90% accuracy.

Methods and Results: During the baserating, William typically interrupted the clinician every 30 sec. He was initially asked to speak only when told "It is your turn to talk." Clinician gave William his turn every 1 min or so. William also was taught to say "It is your turn to talk" when he had spoken for a minute or so. If he did not, he was asked to stop at the end of a sentence. The prompt "It is your turn to talk" was withdrawn in the latter training sessions. If he interrupted, a hand signal to stop was given. This signal also was faded. In the last four sessions, a variable time interval of 1 to 3 min. of talking before allowing the conversational partner to take turns was allowed.

William learned to take conversational turns. On a final probe with no verbal or manual prompt, he took turns on the variable time schedule of one to three minutes of talking with 90% accuracy. Occasionally, he exceeded the range but appropriately.

A final spontaneous language sample was analyzed to determine the need for further clinical services. The analysis revealed an essentially normal language use. Therefore, it is recommended that William be dismissed from treatment.

_____

Noah Webster, B.A.
Student Clinician

_____

Lakshmi Shanker, Ph.D., CCC-SP
Speech-Language Pathologist and Clinical Supervisor

C.4. PROGRESS REPORT: *VOICE TREATMENT*

SIERA SPEECH AND HEARING CENTER
CLOVIS, CA
PROGRESS REPORT

NAME:	**FILE NUMBER:**
BIRTHDATE:	**DIAGNOSIS:** Voice Disorder
ADDRESS:	**DATE OF REPORT:**
CITY:	**PERIOD COVERED:**
TELEPHONE NUMBER:	**CLINICIAN:**

Roshana Hersh, a 21-year-old female college student was seen at the Siera Speech and Hearing Center on March 10, 1993 for a voice evaluation. The evaluation suggested a pattern of vocal abuse associated with a persistent hoarseness of voice and low pitch. A treatment program to improve her voice quality was recommended. The assessment report and a description of her treatment program may be found in her clinical file.

TREATMENT TARGETS

Goal 1: Production of clear voice at least 90% of the time Roshana speaks by reducing the hoarseness of voice

> Objective 1a. Reduced amount of talking over the phone.

> Objective 1b. Reduced amount of shouting at the school.

Goal 2. Increased vocal pitch

> Objective 2a. Higher pitch at the level of words and phrases.

> Objective 2b. Higher pitch at the level of conversational speech.

TREATMENT PROCEDURES AND RESULTS

Objectives 1a and 1b. During the first week, the durations of Roshana's telephone conversation were baserated. The diary record she kept showed that Roshana spoke between 8 to 10 times over the phone each day and that the duration of her phone calls ranged between 10 to 20 min. Sixty percent of her phone calls typically exceeded 15 min.

During the second week, Roshana was asked to reduce by 10% the amount of telephone conversation time. She continued to record the amount of time she spent talking over the phone. In subsequent weeks, she was asked to progressively decrease the amount of time spent on telephone with a goal of reducing the duration by about 50%.

The frequency of shouting also was similarly baserated. On an average day, she tended to shout 8 to 10 times. Roshana was asked to reduce the frequency of shouting behavior in 10% decrements until the frequency approached zero.

Roshana made excellent progress in reducing the frequency and duration of phone calls and in reducing the frequency of shouting. At the end of the semester, Roshana's phone calls averaged between 3 to 7 min. Only an exceptional phone call exceeded this range. Her shouting behavior was reduced to no more than two per day. According to Roshana, her shouts are not as loud as they use to be.

Objectives 2a and 2b. The Visi-Pitch was used to shape a higher pitch consistent with Roshana's gender and age. The treatment was started at the word and phrase level and moved to conversational speech level.

Roshana's speaking fundamental frequency in the clinic increased from a baserate of 157 Hz to 200 Hz toward the end of the semester. However, she still reports a much lower pitch outside the clinic.

It is recommended that Roshana continue to receive voice therapy next semester. The emphasis should be on generalization and maintenance of appropriate target vocal characteristics in extraclinical situations. Roshana needs training in self-monitoring skills.

Signed:_____

      Pero Boss, B.A.

      Student Clinician

Signed:_____

      Moss Nero, M.A., CCC-SP

      Speech-Language Pathologist and Clinical Supervisor

Date_____

Note to Student Clinicians

Contact your clinic director to find out how progress reports vary in your clinic. Contact a private speech and hearing clinic to find out how clinicians there write progress reports they send to health insurance companies.

C.4.1. PROGRESS REPORTS WRITTEN AS LETTERS

Some progress reports are written in the form of a letter. Such progress reports are necessary when the clinician:

- makes a referral to another professional for continued speech-language services
- makes a referral to a different professional
- makes a claim for payment for services from an agency

C.4.1. PROGRESS REPORT: *WRITTEN AS A LETTER*

**SOUTHERN CALIFORNIA SPEECH AND HEARING CENTER
LONG BEACH, CALIFORNIA**

April 25, 1993

Dr. Kim Yang
Long Beach Neurologists, Inc.
Long Beach, California

RE: Juniper Joginder

Dear Dr. Yang:

I am referring Mr. Joginder, a 57-year-old man, to you for a neurological examination. Mr. Joginder experienced a left hemisphere CVA on February 7, 1991 and was subsequently admitted to St. Thomas Medical Center. On February 12, 1991, he was transferred to Los Angeles Rehabilitation Hospital (LARH) where he received physical therapy, occupational therapy, and speech therapy. A speech-language evaluation was completed at LARH, and was diagnosed with severe receptive and expressive aphasia and severe vocal apraxia. He received speech-language therapy at LARH from February 12, 1991 to May 31, 1991. Mr. Joginder's level of functioning while at LARH would have been documented by them, and you will need to obtain their report for details. Upon his discharge from LARH, Mr. Joginder began receiving speech-language therapy at Southern California Speech and Hearing Center. He has attended therapy twice a week for a total of 60 visits.

Initially, Mr. Joginder's understanding of spoken speech and reading were moderately impaired. These skills are now within normal limits and completely functional.
Mr. Joginder's expressive language was severely impaired. Following the CVA, he was virtually non-verbal except for a few paraphasic utterances. Word retrieval deficits and verbal apraxia were severe. When he began therapy at Southern California Speech and Hearing Center, Mr. Joginder was working on word retrieval, producing multisyllable words (90%), and using multi-syllable words in a variety of target sentence structures (70%). His word retrieval skills have

improved significantly. He currently can cite antonyms or synonyms with 90 to 100% accuracy, provide words when given a description or definition with 90% accuracy, and name pictures with 90 to 100% accuracy. Mr. Joginder can formulate sentences when given a word with 70 to 90% accuracy, answer simple questions with 80 to 90% accuracy, and describe pictures with 90 to 100% accuracy.

Most recently, I have been working with Mr. Joginder's lecture notes. Currently, he can organize and create a written outline on his own. Using his outline, he can now present a 30 to 45 min lecture with 75 to 90% accuracy. He can answer simple questions about the lecture with 70 to 80% accuracy.

Overall, Mr. Joginder has made remarkable progress in all targeted speech-language skills. He has excellent family support. Therefore, it is recommended that he continue to receive speech-language therapy with an emphasis on:

1.   high-level word retrieval skills,

2.   sentence and question formulation,

3.   spontaneous responses to questions,

4.   lecturing skills,

5.   accurate production of "work related vocabulary,"

6.   accurate production of multi-syllable words and words containing difficult blends or sound combinations, and

7.   overall conversational speech skills.

I hope this information is helpful. I look forward to receiving your report on Mr. Joginder. Please contact me if you have questions. Thank you.

Yours sincerely,

_____

Von Tran, M.A., CCC-SP
Speech-Language Pathologist

Note to Student Clinicians

Contact your supervisor and directors of private speech clinics to find out what kinds of letters are typically sent to government agencies that reimburse clinicians for speech, language, and hearing services. Some agencies may use printed forms. Obtain samples of such forms.

C.5. PRACTICE IN WRITING PROGRESS REPORTS

C.5. PROGRESS REPORT: *TREATMENT OF STUTTERING*

UNIVERSITY SPEECH AND HEARING CLINIC
FREEMONT UNIVERSITY
VALLEYVILLE, CALIFORNIA

PROGRESS REPORT

NAME: Winston Churchill   **FILE NUMBER:**

BIRTHDATE: **DIAGNOSIS:** Stuttering

ADDRESS: **DATE OF REPORT:**

CITY: **PERIOD COVERED:**

TELEPHONE NUMBER: **CLINICIAN:**

CLINIC SCHEDULE

Sessions per week_____   Clock hr of individual therapy:_____

Length of sessions:_____   Clock hr of group therapy:_____

Number of clinic visits:_____   Total clock hr of therapy:_____

Data Sheet	
Winston Churchill, 22 yrs.	Who, how old, came to which clinic, and with what problem?
Stuttering	
Two conversational speech samples (9 and 11% dysfluency rate) One reading sample (22% dysfluency rate)	(Summarize the assessment data in one or two sentences.)
Received treatment for stuttering for one semester	Received treatment for what and for how long?

C.5. PROGRESS REPORT: *TREATMENT OF STUTTERING*

Write your report. Invent information as needed.

Who, how old, came to which clinic, and with what problem?

(Summarize the assessment data in one or two sentences.)

Received treatment for what and for how long?

Data Sheet	
	SUMMARY OF TREATMENT (L1H)
Normal-sounding fluency in natural settings with less than 5% dysfluency rate (or any other objectives you select)	**Final Treatment Objectives? (L2H)**
Gentle phonatory onset Airflow management Rate reduction through syllable stretching	**Treatment Targets? (L2H)**
Two conversational speech baselines of 10 and 11%	**Baselines?**
Modeling and imitation; controlled utterances; movement from words to phrases and conversational speech; verbal praise; corrective feedback for mismanagement of the target behaviors or for dysfluencies	**Treatment Procedures? (L2H)**
	Establishment
Twice-a-week sessions of 50 minutes	**Training**
	PROGRESS (L1H)
Good progress: Dysfluency rates reduced to 5% in conversational probes in the clinic; about 6 to 7% at home	**How was progress measured? (Probe and other procedures)**
	What were the results?
Continued treatment recommended to further reduce the dysfluencies and to initiate a maintenance program.	**Recommendations**
	Signature lines
	Student Clinician
	Supervisor

Write your report. Invent information as needed.

SUMMARY OF
TREATMENT
(L1H)

Final Treatment
Objectives? **(L2H)**

Treatment Targets?
(L2H)

Baselines?

Treatment Procedures?
(L2H)

Establishment

Training

PROGRESS
(L2H)

How was progress
measured? (Probe and
other procedures)

What were the results?

Recommendations

Signature lines

Student Clinician

Supervisor

C.5. PROGRESS REPORT: *TREATMENT OF AN ARTICULATION DISORDER*

UNIVERSITY SPEECH AND HEARING CENTER
BLOOM, ILLINOIS
PROGRESS REPORT

NAME: FILE NUMBER:

BIRTHDATE: DIAGNOSIS: Articulation Disorder

ADDRESS: DATE OF REPORT:

CITY: PERIOD COVERED:

TELEPHONE NUMBER: CLINICIAN:

CLINIC SCHEDULE

Sessions per week:_____   Clock hr of individual therapy:_____

Length of session:_____   Clock hr of group therapy:_____

Number of clinic visits:_____ Total clock hr of therapy:_____

Data Sheet

Jimmy Jones, 6 yrs.

Articulation disorder
Omissions of initial and final /k, s, t, p, b/

No prior treatment

Who, how old, came to which clinic and with what problem?
(Summarize the assessment data in one or two sentences.)
Received treatment for what and for how long?

C.5. PROGRESS REPORT: *TREATMENT OF AN ARTICULATION DISORDER*

Write your report. Invent information as needed.

Who, how old, came to which clinic and with what problem?

(Summarize the assessment data in one or two sentences.)

Received treatment for what and for how long?

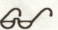

Data Sheet	
	PROGRESS (L1H)
Teaching the phonemes in word initial positions	Objective 1 (L2H)
Baserated Modeling, imitation, successive approximation, differential verbal feedback Training criterion (90% correct) Probe: 95% correct	Methods and Results (L2H)
Teaching the phonemes in word final positions	Objective 2 (L2H)
Baserated Modeling, imitation, successive approximation, differential verbal feedback Training criterion (90% correct)	Methods and Results (L2H)
Production of phonemes in phrases and sentences Probe: 95% correct	Objective 3 (L2H)
Productions in phrases, sentences, and conversational speech reinforced Probe: 95% correct	Methods and Results
Development of a home treatment program for maintenance	Objective 4 (L2H)
Training the father in evoking and reinforcing the phonemes in conversational speech at home Probe: 80% correct	Methods and Results (L2H)
	Recommendations
Additional treatment	Signature lines
Your name	Student Clinician
Your Supervisor's name	Supervisor

Write your report. Invent information as needed.	
	PROGRESS (L1H)
	Objective 1 (L2H)
	Methods and Results (L2H)
	Objective 2 (L2H)
	Methods and Results (L2H)
	Objective 3 (L2H)
	Methods and Results
	Objective 4 (L2H)
	Methods and Results (L2H)
	Recommendations
	Signature lines
	Student Clinician
	Supervisor

C.5. PROGRESS REPORT: *TREATMENT OF LANGUAGE DISORDER*

UNIVERSITY SPEECH AND HEARING CENTER
BELLVIEW UNIVERSITY
BELLVIEW, WASHINGTON

Client: Date of Birth:

Period Covered: Clinician:

CLINIC SCHEDULE

Session per week:_____   Clock hr of individual therapy:_____

Length of session:_____   Clock hr of group therapy:_____

Number of clinic visits:_____   Total clock hr of therapy:_____

PROGRESS REPORT

NAME: FILE NUMBER:

BIRTHDATE: DIAGNOSIS:

ADDRESS: DATE OF REPORT:

CITY: PERIOD COVERED:

TELEPHONE NUMBER: CLINICIAN:

Data Sheet	
Tanya Tucker, 6 yrs.	Who, how old, came to which clinic, and with what problem?
Language disorders. Does not produce ing, auxiliary is, regular and irregular plurals. regular past tense, prepositions, and pronouns	(Summarize the assessment data in one or two sentences.)
Two semester's of treatment on vocabulary expansion	Received treatment for what and for how long?

C.5. PROGRESS REPORT: *TREATMENT OF LANGUAGE DISORDER*

Write your report. Invent information as needed.

Who, how old, came to which clinic, and with what problem?

(Summarize the assessment data in one or two sentences.)

Received treatment for what and for how long?

Data Sheet

	SUMMARY OF TREATMENT (L1H)

ing, auxiliary *is*, and regular plural in sentences

	Target Behaviors (L2H)

| | Performance Criterion? |

Ninety percent correct in conversational speech

| | Methods and Results? (L2H) |

Twenty senteces for each target. Baserate: 0 to 10%

| | Baselines? |

Initially, training with discrete trials; finally, training in conversational speech

| | How was progress measured? (Probe and other procedures) |

Minimally 10 probe sentences

In conversational speech:
ing, 90% correct

| | What were the results? |

auxiliary *is*, 70% correct

regular plural, 80%

Continued treatment on the auxiliary and the plural morpheme
Training on additional grammatic morphemes

| | Recommendations |

Your name

| | Signature lines |

Your supervisor's name

| | Student Clinician |

| | Supervisor |

Write your report. Invent information as needed.

SUMMARY OF
TREATMENT
(L1H)

Target Behaviors
(L2H)

Performance
Criterion?

Methods and
Results?
(L2H)

Baselines?

How was progress
measured? (Probe
and other
procedures)

What were the
results?

Recommendations

Signature lines

Student Clinician

Supervisor

C.5. PROGRESS REPORT: *VOICE DISORDER*

THE SUNSHINE SPEECH AND HEARING CENTER
ZINGSVILLE, VERMONT

NAME: FILE NUMBER:

BIRTHDATE: DIAGNOSIS: Voice Disorder

ADDRESS: DATE OF REPORT:

CITY: PERIOD COVERED:

TELEPHONE NUMBER: CLINICIAN:

Data Sheet

Raj Mohan, 35 yrs. High school teacher	Who, how old, came to which clinic, and with what problem?
Inadequate loudness; voice too soft; students complain; his voice gets tired; ENT report negative; no contraindications for voice therapy	(Summarize the assessment data in one or two sentences.)
No prior treatment	Received treatment for what and for how long?

C.5. PROGRESS REPORT: *VOICE DISORDER*

Write your report. Invent information as needed.

Who, how old, came to which clinic, and with what problem?

(Summarize the assessment data in one or two sentences.)

Received treatment for what and for how long?

Data Sheet	
	SUMMARY OF TREATMENT (L1H)
Increase vocal loudness; adequate loudness for classroom teaching as rated by the clinician and his students across a minimum of four teaching sessions.	Objectives? (L2H) (The same as treatment targets)
Student reactions to be probed across four lecture hours on 4 days	Performance Criterion?
	Methods and Results? (L2H)
The clinician's and students' rating of loudness on a 5-point rating scale in three class periods Recording the frequency of student requests for louder speech	Baselines?
	Establishment
Verbal reinforcement of progressively louder speech Masking noise to increase vocal intensity (Lombard effect) Visi-Pitch feedback to shape progressively louder voice	How was progress measured? (Probe and other procedures)
Adequate loudness as rated in the classroom across three lecture periods on separate days	What were the results?
Schedule a follow-up in 3 months to assess maintenance of adequate loudness	Recommendations
Your name	Signature lines
	Student Clinician
Supervisor's name	Supervisor

Write your report. Invent information as needed

SUMMARY OF
TREATMENT
(L1H)

Objectives? (L2H)
(The same as
treatment targets)

Performance
Criterion?

Methods and
Results?
(L2H)

Baselines?

Establishment

How was progress
measured? (Probe
and other
procedures)

What were the
results?

Recommendations

Signature lines

Student Clinician

Supervisor

C.5. PROGRESS REPORT: *WRITTEN AS A LETTER*

On the next page, write a letter to a speech-language pathologist describing *the progress a 7-year-old child with an articulation disorder* made under your treatment. Invent information as needed.

C.5. PROGRESS REPORT: *WRITTEN AS A LETTER*

The name of your clinic (L1H)

Date

Describe the child and his or her problem.

Give a brief history.

Summarize your assessment.

Summarize your treatment targets or objectives.

Summarize your treatment procedures.

Summarize the results or the progress

State your recommendations.

Sign your name.

Note to Student Clinicians

Select a case with aphasia and write a progress report on treating naming problems. Use the format shown on the previous pages.

C.6. PROFESSIONAL CORRESPONDENCE

Correspondence with clients, parents of clients, teachers, medical and other specialists is an important part of clinical duties. The letters a professional person about his or her services reflect training and competence. A well written letter may inspire confidence in a clinician. A clumsy letter may detract potential clients from the clinician's services. Professional letters should look good as well. This means that they should be on a letterhead printed on 25% cotton bond paper.

Professional letters should be:

- Accurate

    Give correct information based only on your observations.

- Brief and to the point

    Those who receive your letter may be busy people. So be brief and give only the most essential information.

- Suitable to the person receiving it

    If you write a letter to another professional who is expected to know your technical terms, use those terms. If the recipient is expected not to know your technical terms, use general terms.

Variety of Professional letters include:

- *Thank you* letters written to persons or agencies that referred a client
- Letters that describe treatment progress (usually sent to a referring or paying agency)
- Letters that make a referral to another professional

C.6. A *THANK YOU* LETTER

CALIFORNIA STATE UNIVERSITY, FRESNO
SPEECH AND HEARING CLINIC
FRESNO, CA 93740

September 5, 1993

Dr. John Lamp
Lamp Pediatric Medical Group
0405 E. Marks
Fresno, CA 98728

Dear Dr. Lamp:

Thank you for referring Eric Martinez to the Speech and Hearing Clinic at California State University, Fresno for stuttering evaluation and treatment. We evaluated Eric's speech and language on September 2, 1993. Eric's mother brought him to the clinic. Mrs. Martinez brought a tape recorded speech sample from home which was analyzed as part of the evaluation.

Results of the assessment revealed a moderate to severe stuttering with a dysfluency rate of 15 to 20%. His stuttering is characterized by sound repetitions, intralexical pauses, interjections, and pauses. A few articulation errors were noted, but did not interfere with speech intelligibility. Receptive and expressive language were judged age-appropriate.

It was recommended that Eric receive treatment for his stuttering. He is currently enrolled at the CSUF Speech and Hearing Clinic. In December, we will let you know about Eric's progress in treatment. If you have questions, please contact the clinic at 555-2142.

Sincerely,

_____

Athena Bacona, B.A.
Student Clinician

_____

Winthrop Venkat, M.A., CCC-SP
Supervisor, Speech-Language Pathologist

C.6. A *REFERRAL* LETTER

SUNSHINE SPEECH AND HEARING CLINIC
SUNSHINE, MN

September 25, 1993

Kristen Goodnow, M.D.
25 E. Cloudy, Suite 301
Sunshine, MN 00501

Dear Dr. Goodnow:

I evaluated John Jacobs, a 42-year-old man for a voice disorder on September 22, 1993. Mr. Jacobs reported that his voice is "too rough" and that he wanted treatment. He works in noisy construction areas. His history suggests chronic hoarseness and occasional pain in his laryngeal area. My evaluation indicates a harsh and breathy voice with frequent pitch breaks. He cannot sustain phonation. His speech intensity drops at the end of his sentences.

I am referring Mr. Jacobs to you for a laryngeal examination. I have enclosed a copy of my evaluation report. If there are no contraindications, I plan to start a voice treatment program after your examination. Therefore, please send me a copy of your report. Also, please contact me if you have questions. Thank you for your help.

Yours sincerely,

Sylvia Rodriguez, Ph.D., CCC-SP
Speech-Language Pathologist

Note to Student Clinicians

Contact your clinic secretary to find out about *thank you* letters written to other professionals.
Also, find out about other kinds of letters your clinic sends out.

C.7. PRACTICE IN WRITING PROFESSIONAL CORRESPONDENCE

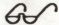

C.7. A *THANK YOU* LETTER

On the next page, write a *thank you* letter to a neurologist who has referred to you *a patient with aphasia.*

C.7. A *THANK YOU* LETTER

The name of your clinic
(**L1H**)

Date

The name, title, and address of the person receiving the letter.

Describe the child and his or her problem.

Summarize your assessment.

State your recommendations.

Sign your name.

C.7. A *REFERRAL* LETTER

On the next page, write A *Referral* letter to a reading specialist to whom you refer a child. Assume that you are treating this child for an oral language disorder and that he or she needs treatment for reading problems.

C.7. A *REFERRAL* LETTER

The name of your clinic (L1H)

Date

The name, title, and address of the person receiving the letter.

Describe the child and his or her problem.

Give a brief history.

Summarize your assessment.

Summarize your treatment targets, procedures, and results.

State your recommendations.

Sign your name.

Note to Student Writers

Please go back and check the entire book to make sure that you have completed all writing assignments. The only method of learning to write well is to write and rewrite. Complete the unfinished assignments.

DETAILED TABLE OF CONTENTS